To Theo,

A beautiful spirit who
works miracles, and who
I hope to meet one day.

Affectionately,

Fay

5/11/'10

SILENT ENEMY

*Environmental Illness and
One Woman's Search for a Cure*

Faye Hueston

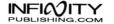
INFINITY
PUBLISHING.COM

ISBN 0-7414-5121-2

Published by:

INFIᐤITY
PUBLISHING.COM

1094 New DeHaven Street, Suite 100
West Conshohocken, PA 19428-2713
Info@buybooksontheweb.com
www.buybooksontheweb.com
Toll-free (877) BUY BOOK
Local Phone (610) 941-9999
Fax (610) 941-9959

Printed in the United States of America

Published March 2010

In memory of Rachel Carson,
Who sounded the warning,

And of Dr. Max Gerson,
Who provided the cure.

Rarely has anything been accomplished except by the genius of a single man, fighting against the crowd.

Voltaire

Man has lost the capacity to foresee and to forestall. He will end by destroying the earth.

Albert Schweitzer

WARNING

The author is not a licensed physician and does not present her experiences with medical treatment as a guide for patients in need of care. Do not attempt self-diagnosis or initiate treatment based on the content of this book. The experiences related here are unique to the author and are not offered as a substitute for a licensed physician's in-person medical evaluation, diagnosis, and recommended treatment.

PROLOGUE

Some years ago, while living in London, I became unaccountably ill. A mysterious process seemed to be at work within my body, undermining the vigorous health I enjoyed throughout most of my life. This slow, imperceptible slide into infirmity alarmed me, for I was ill-prepared for sickness.

Raised as a Christian Scientist by my adoptive mother, I grew up in a Hollywood home that was affluent, pious, and teetotal. Believing all illness to be a mental "belief" we saw no doctors, nor were there any medicines in our medicine cabinets. The only cure for a headache or a heart attack was prayer.

My adoptive father did not share our religion, although he was sympathetic toward it because of his deep mistrust of quacks—the term with which he dismissed the doctors he never saw. While the connection between our faith and our genes may have been merely fortuitous, my parents, my adoptive brother, and I rejoiced in excellent health.

In 1963, constant prayer notwithstanding, my first serious illness brought me close to death. Saved at the eleventh hour by a doctor with antibiotics, and disillusioned with God and Mary Baker Eddy, both of whom I felt had let me down, I left the church. What I did not know was that my body still harbored the seeds of a future struggle—seeds that were to germinate for the next sixteen years.

I do not deny that spiritual healing occurs or that symptoms can, on occasion, be psychosomatically produced. My story, however, concerns a more prevalent case of illness in which prayer proves ineffectual and symptoms thought to be psychosomatic in origin, when correctly diagnosed, are found to have an environmental cause.

As invasive chemicals multiply with frightening complexity in the world, they bring new and graver challenges for human health and survival. We are faced with an increasingly drug- and technology-oriented medicine that is ill-equipped to deal with the subtle nature of environmental illness. We have merely to consider the levels of pollution in our food, our water, and in the air we breathe, to realize the harm we are inflicting—not only on ourselves, but on this fragile planet, our earthly home.

During the years of declining health, when no one knew what was wrong with me, I thought I must be the only person in the world so strangely afflicted. Yet something told me this could not be true. I was neither sinful enough nor saintly enough to be singled out for some exotic torment. After my condition was diagnosed and the road to recovery began, I determined that if I should be healed, an account of my journey might help others who find themselves in a similar predicament.

Throughout this experience I kept a diary. Begun for the purpose of recording my dreams, some of which were proving to be precognitive, it became instead a record of the symptoms, setbacks and fears that accompanied the long, discouraging search for a cure.

The following pages are a chronicle distilled from that journey, which finally led to the unorthodox therapy that saved my life. It is in the hope of sparing others the same suffering and wasted years that I have written this book.

CHAPTER ONE

Square my trial to my proportioned strength.
—Milton

I sensed something was wrong the moment I surfaced from the anesthetic. The feeling of a tight band across my forehead and an acid crawling under my scalp, together with the pain that ran from a hip down one leg, were new acquisitions. It was my fifth operation within a year—this last to remove a silicone breast implant, following a mastectomy for cancer three months before.

Within weeks of the implant's insertion my breast began to swell. Assuming the cause to be an infection, the surgeon prescribed an antibiotic. I had been given so many antibiotics by then I was loath to take more, but having transferred my faith in God to faith in doctors, I lacked the courage to question higher authority.

When the first course proved ineffective, my surgeon prescribed a stronger, broad-spectrum course of the drugs, but this failed as well. By the time he proposed a third course, my breast felt like a balloon about to burst and I demanded the implant be removed. A tissue sample was sent to the lab to see if a culture could be grown, but the report came back negative.

"Why, then, did my body reject the implant?" I asked the surgeon.

"I don't know," he replied. "It shouldn't have rejected it, because silicone is inert matter."

Little was known in the 1970s about the effect of silicone in the body, even when it was "safely" enclosed in a breast form. It didn't occur to me that the many drugs I was given

1

that year—tranquilizers, anesthetics, painkillers, and six courses of antibiotics—might have contributed to the rejection. I only knew that between the time I entered the operating theater and the moment I regained consciousness in my room, something happened to my body that had nothing to do with the surgery on my breast.

Too drugged to think clearly, I assumed the symptoms would disappear, but they didn't. The painful sciatica lasted for almost a year. A friend who had been a nurse told me that patients were sometimes handled roughly when under anesthesia and being transported from the operating theatre to their rooms.

"It's not uncommon for minor injuries to occur," she said. "It's also not generally known that medical students are allowed to perform pelvic examinations on anesthetized women."

"Pelvic exams! Without our knowledge or consent?"

"That's right. Of course, you'd have a job trying to prove it in court, or to prove a minor injury such as yours. You can't touch the unions—or the doctors for that matter. They all close ranks."

In the weeks that followed I became aware of a slight burning sensation under my scalp, as though a mild acid was spreading under the skin. Months later, my hairline appeared to be receding. When the condition continued, I consulted my National Health Service (NHS) doctor—a cold, remote man I had met only once before, when my sixteen-year-old daughter came down with the flu.

"Well?" he said as I entered, lifting his eyes from the papers on his desk. It was his only greeting. I ran through my repertoire of symptoms, while he listened with all the interest of a bored mortician. When I described the peculiar sensation under my skin, he rose and made a cursory examination of my scalp. Finding no visible anomaly, he pronounced my symptoms psychosomatic.

"I know there's nothing you can see," I protested. "That's what's so puzzling."

He studied me for a moment. "Have you thought of seeing a psychiatrist about this?" he asked.

"Why, no," I said, taken aback.

"I suggest that would be your best step," he advised and returned to his desk. Since the visit appeared to be over, I apologized for wasting his time and left.

Dismissed by the National Health, I turned to the private sector—a quest that took me through some of the costliest consulting rooms in London, without bringing me any closer to a diagnosis or cure. At least the doctors I paid privately were too polite to say they thought I was mad. Instead, they fobbed me off with useless ointments, practiced smiles, and healthy bills.

A Sloane Street trichologist with impeccable manners examined my scalp and assured me the receding hair would grow back in the spring. Weeks later, a Mayfair specialist informed me it would never grow back. The only point on which the two experts agreed was that neither had a cure to offer.

A third deity—a diminutive dermatologist in Harley Street, with a large Arab clientele—had the honesty, or the chutzpah, to admit that no one really knows what causes hair to fall out. For this wisdom I received a bill larger than those presented by the other two. What a doddle this skin game is, I thought; all you need to charge the earth for your ignorance is an expensive education.

Weary of doctors who had no time for difficult conditions—not even as a challenge on which to sharpen their skills—I turned to the alternative field. The 1970s were a time of bold new approaches to health in holistic medicine. Disciplines such as Silva Mind Control and the Simontons' visualization technique were stressing the integration of mind, body, and spirit in the healing process.

It was the ME generation, before new-age became old hat—when it was wrong to be judgmental and nothing was either right or wrong, since actions could be whatever you wanted them to be. Embracing it all, I attended seminars given by self-styled gurus who jetted the world promising instant nirvana (for a price), joined consciousness-raising groups whose leaders tried to bludgeon me into Enlightenment, and met a few self-effacing souls along the way, who encouraged me to find the light within.

During a transpersonal psychology workshop, we were given a guided meditation that involved climbing a mountain, at the top of which we would meet a wise old man who would tell us something we needed to know. The mountain appeared quite readily behind closed eyelids, rising from a meadow of yellow jonquils, its peak bathed in the violet hues of a setting sun.

Athrob with expectation I reached the summit, but found no wise old man there ready to counsel me. I waited for him to appear, until I heard the leader's voice instructing us to bring our consciousness back to the room. When we all had returned from our inner journeys, the leader invited us to share the message that each had received. To my chagrin, I was the only one to whom no wise old man appeared. I felt mortified, rebuffed, my unworthiness confirmed.

A year later, the same meditation was given in a different workshop and again, I found myself on that mountaintop—alone, waiting, and close to tears. Eventually, a wise old woman appeared, but if she told me something I needed to know, I forgot it on the way down.

I tried Transcendental Meditation, but fared no better. Thoughts flitted and strayed, were brought under control, then scampered away again. Unwanted tunes kept playing in my head, like musical tinnitus. My chattering mind could not be stilled.

Inspired by a book on self-healing through visualization, I tried to imagine my white blood cells mobilizing and destroying the condition that was undermining my health. But the condition had no name and no known cause, hence no image that I could visualize, so I abandoned the effort.

Turning to the more practical end of the alternative field, I tried homeopathy, reflexology, osteopathy, iridology, kinesiology, acupuncture and herbal remedies—each for a period long enough to determine its efficacy for me. On the whole, the practitioners I met were men and women of transparent dedication, each believing that his or her patch of the holistic field was the answer to most, if not all of the body's ills.

"Your third chakra is unbalanced," said one therapist.

"What does that mean?"

"It means your stomach, liver, and nervous systems are out of balance. You need to be more grounded. And your yin-yang energy needs balancing as well."

To be sure, there were a few charlatans along the way, but they were as easy to spot as their orthodox brethren. Yet, wide though my net had been cast, by 1979 I was no better; in fact I was getting worse. The fault, however, lay not with the therapies, for if they did not help, neither did they harm. It was simply that they had evolved at a time when mankind was cooperating with nature instead of trying to subdue her—a time when the world was a gentler and purer place than it has since become.

Sadly, their methods were no match for the invisible enemy that was insinuating itself, slowly and silently, into every cell of my being.

CHAPTER TWO

I am the self-consumer of my woes.
                —John Clare

As my health continued to decline my sense of isolation increased. It was as if I had been drawn into some dark wood where there was no path, no guide, and where no one had gone before. In *The Masks of God,* Joseph Campbell paraphrases Dante's "adventure of the dark wood" as the psychological journey that occurs in the middle of life. Symbolically, it represents crucifixion, death, and the descent into hell, followed by the passage through purgatory that leads, ultimately, to paradise and the adventurer's return to service in the world. As I was fast approaching the descent-into-hell phase, the prospect of paradise seemed to be lost indeed.

In January 1980, I applied to the NHS to change my general practitioner. The new doctor—a youngish woman with short-cropped brown hair and a brisk, impersonal manner—listened as I explained that my problems began three years earlier.

"... And still, no one can determine the cause of my symptoms," I concluded.

"Which are?"

I gave her a well-rehearsed rundown of the pincushion scalp, the sense of a band tightening around my head and the sick-all-over-feeling I woke up with each morning. From the expression on her face I might have been addressing a sphinx.

"Yes," she said, "I'm familiar with these symptoms. They're emotionally caused. Have you thought of seeing a psychiatrist?"

I blinked. This woman knew nothing about me. She hadn't even received my records from the former GP, whatever *they* contained. Yet within minutes of meeting me, she concluded that my symptoms were imaginary—as though incipient male-pattern baldness in a healthy, middle-aged woman could be emotionally caused. If that were so, by forty we would all be bald.

I returned home more discouraged than ever. It wasn't only that no one understood what was wrong with me; it was that no one cared enough to *want* to understand. Of course it is easier for the busy doctor to consign a peculiar patient to the ministrations of a psychiatrist, even though it was not so long ago that psychiatry itself was viewed with sniffy disdain. No matter; if the answer eludes pathology, the psychosomatic excuse can always be trotted out (Freud has a lot to answer for!). And if the patient, on hearing the word "psychosomatic" for the tenth time, feels the teeniest urge to scream—well, that just proves the case, doesn't it?

No doubt there are those whose illnesses are emotionally caused, but I was not one of them. Raised in a religion that views sickness as "a manifestation of erroneous thinking," I was more inclined to deny its reality than create it. Yet, even if we are the author of our woes, by what process does the mind create unwanted illness in the body? If disease is so easily acquired against our will, why is the mind so impotent when seeking consciously to be well? I put this question to a number of practitioners, but answer came there none.

As for the cause being emotional, I had never felt more emotionally serene. I had moved to London in 1970 after a divorce in Paris; I had two young daughters I adored and a relationship with someone who shared my love of literature and music. Moreover, with no financial worries, thanks to the bequest of my adoptive parents, I had time to work on a book I was writing about my adoptive experience.

Physically, however, my problems were multiplying. Arthritis was stiffening my joints and interfering with the yoga I had practiced for seven years. When I rose from my desk my knees crunched like gravel, and when I turned my head to the left my neck felt like a block of grinding pain. Rhinitis and hay fever, too, were recurring miseries.

At night, I woke with a pounding headache or a teeth-chattering chill that sent me scurrying for a sweater, even in summer. The panic attacks and sudden flushes I assumed to be harbingers of menopause—of which as yet there was no sign. Moreover, the sickly flushes did not conform to those described by a menopausal friend, whose nighttime sweats and fevers were causing her a different kind of distress.

My flushes were more like a "chaos of the mind"—the phrase Lord Byron used to describe his spells of manic depression. They began near the base of my spine and rose in a sickening wave to my head, where they imploded in my brain like a silent madness. It was as though I was losing my mind, while remaining sane enough to feel each step of the disintegrating process. What made the waves so frightening was the loss of parameter—the sense of there being no edge to hold onto.

As my benighted body relinquished one aspect of health after another, I felt betrayed—the way a great beauty must feel betrayed when her perfect face begins to wrinkle and sag. There was also the effect my condition was having on the relationship with my daughters. Because my symptoms were sporadic, with no visible cause, Kate and Amy viewed my claims of illness as suspect and me as the most tiresome of mothers.

"I don't believe you're really sick," said fourteen-year-old Amy, observing me in bed with a crippling migraine.

"All you do is go to healers and doctors and have operations," said sixteen-year-old Kate, the day I came home from having the implant removed.

And who could blame them? The search for health had taken over my life.

In the silent war being waged within my body, an attack could come at any moment. It could manifest as a tingling in my feet, or a sudden fever in the head, or my heart would begin to fibrillate, as though it was plugged into a generator that could not be switched off. I was also becoming hypersensitive to noise. The slam of a door or the sound of a pneumatic drill on the pavement outside—even the cry of a child in the street below, affected me like an assault on my central nervous system.

George Eliot, in *Middlemarch,* observes that "if we had a keen vision and feeling of all ordinary human life, it would be like hearing the grass grow and the squirrel's heart beat, and we should die of that roar which lies on the other side of silence." There were times when the inrush of sensory data was like that silent roar—inaudible to others, yet overwhelming me with its noise.

One could hardly devise a more diabolic torment than one in which the victim is subject to forces no one can see, with symptoms for which no cause can be found, while appearing outwardly to be perfectly well. Such a condition, if imposed on a criminal, would be deemed cruel and inhuman punishment. Who had I wronged? What had I done that I should be punished so?

By May 1980, a year of acupuncture had failed to relieve my headaches or hay fever. Homeopathy and herbal treatment failed as well. But why? Others were helped by these therapies, why not me? At times, my naturally curly hair would go limp for weeks before regaining its normal texture and curl. There *had* to be a connection with the sense of an acid spreading under my scalp.

Advice came from every quarter, all of it well-meaning, most of it wrong. One doctor told me my problem was hormonal, another said it was too much acid, while a third diagnosed an infection. The rest insisted it was all in my mind. One healer told me, "You're blocked." Another said, "You're too open." A third said, "Your aura is as full of holes as Swiss cheese." At the end of three years I had seen

9

so many doctors, healers, and therapists, I wouldn't have known who to credit if I got better or what to blame if I got worse.

As the symptoms increased my frustration grew, for I knew they were not psychosomatic; they were *somatopsychic,* the body influencing the brain. I knew this because my body kept telling me they were and I had learned to listen to its still small voice.

Often, during this period, a moment from childhood appeared in my mind's eye—like a loop of film playing the same scene over and over. I saw myself at the age of eight or nine, running across the lawn of our Beverly Hills home and thinking, *How strong I am! I shall always be strong and healthy like this. Why does anyone have to be ill? If I'm ever sick, I shall simply will myself to be well!* Conscious only of health, I took it to be a legacy for life. Nothing could harm me, I was invincible!

Such arrogance of the fittest must have angered the gods, for one bent down just then and whispered in my ear, "Mark well this moment, child, and the health of which you are now so certain, for the memory may return one day to haunt you."

The merest blink of a moment—as evanescent as a thousand moments more important and long forgotten, yet it embedded itself in my mind, like a fly trapped in amber, waiting to mock me now—now that I knew how impotent is the will in the face of illness.

CHAPTER THREE

Dreams are letters from the unconscious.
—C.G. Jung

In December 1980, the therapist to whom I submitted my arthritic joints for a monthly kneading advised me to walk for an hour each day. "Take strong, purposeful strides," he ordered. "Sitting too long at your desk is part of the problem." So I strode through a nearby park, savoring the snow and the stillness, but at the end of three months my legs were no better. Something unwonted kept sapping my strength.

To be afflicted with the infirmities of age while still relatively young seemed an egregious affront. There were things I meant to do with my life—productive, outgoing things, such as writing and being of service to others in some way—not waste it in this constant preoccupation with my body. There had to be an explanation for what was happening to me, if only to prove wrong those all-knowing doctors who told me my symptoms were self-induced or all in the mind. How did they know? How could they tell if they weren't living in my skin, if they couldn't feel what *I* was feeling?

By April 1981, I was dragging myself out of bed in the mornings, feeling ancient and feeble and depressed. Hobbling about on aching feet, I went to see a foot reflexologist I knew who lived in a third-floor walk-up off Bayswater Road. Too weak to skip up the stairs as before, I pulled myself up by the handrail, step by slow, painful step, my strong ex-figure skater's thighs as weak as spent rubber bands.

A year had passed since I'd last seen Joe and now, stretched out on his bed with one aching foot in his lap, I said, "I hope *you* can tell me, Joe, what is happening to my body." For several moments he dug at my big toe with an iron thumb, while I dug my fingers into the bedspread to keep from howling.

"Your adrenals are completely drained," he said.

"What does that mean?"

"I'm not sure. Have you been under any stress lately?"

"I've scarcely been without it for the past three years," I answered, with a hollow laugh. "But I don't believe in stress as a causative agent, Joe. We're all under stress of one sort or another, aren't we?"

"Well, something is stressing your body," he said. "The trouble is in your lower spine."

"Then what can it be?" I persisted, yearning for an answer, *any* answer. "I've never had back pain and stress alone can't explain this slow wasting away of my strength."

Joe prodded other points on my foot.

"Are there any stressors in your personal life, perhaps?"

"None," I replied. Indeed, my life had never been happier. My daughters were both at boarding school by then (their choice, not mine), and with my boyfriend, Tony, I was enjoying London's lavish offerings of concerts, opera and theatre. In fact, the only stress in my life was being told by doctors that my symptoms were psychosomatic and I needed to see a psychiatrist.

It was during this period that on the night of April 12th, 1981, I had a dream of such transcendent imagery it changed forever my sense of this waking world as the only reality. I suspect that to each of us is granted, if only once in a lifetime, an intimation of something beyond the now that we know—some hint that the world in which we find ourselves is not all there is. In whatever form the glimpse is given, once experienced, our sense of existence can never again be the same.

The dream—although it was more than a dream—began in the waiting room of a doctor or healer. I'm not sure which, for I have no recollection of seeing the practitioner. The next thing I recalled on waking was leaving his or her office by a different door and walking down a gray corridor that led to the street.

As I stepped onto the sidewalk I looked down—and found that I could see right through the pavement into its transparent depths. Tiny points of light were darting and dancing in the velvety blackness beneath my feet. It was as if I had stepped from a dull, two-dimensional world, into one in which every atom and particle could be seen through the permeable solidity of structure.

Astonished, I raised my eyes and saw that everything around me—trees, houses, the world—was suffused with a golden light unlike any I had seen on earth. It did not merely illumine, it permeated creation with a pellucid, numinous glow. The surfaces of things had thinned and I could see right through them, into their very essence.

"Oh!" I heard myself gasp, *"This* is reality!" I had never seen it before, yet I recognized it instantly—as though from some far memory predating my existence. Engulfed in a kind of cosmic homesickness, I yearned to share the vision with someone, for, strangely, there were no people in this wondrous landscape.

I rushed back to the waiting room—hoping, for no rational reason, to find my daughter, Kate, there, but the room was empty and appeared even bleaker after that crystalline world outside. As I stood there, crestfallen, a silent voice said, "You don't understand. The vision can't be shared. You must experience it alone."

For a moment I felt bereft. But then, fearing the vision had vanished because I turned away from it, I hurried outside—and it was still there, pulsing and shimmering, a transparent world glowing with incandescent beauty.

In May, as my condition worsened, I went to see a Scottish healer I knew, who was on one of his periodic visits south of the border.

I met Bruce MacManaway shortly after moving to England, when I attended one of his week-end seminars. Tall and imposing, a former major in the British Army, he taught subjects such as healing, extrasensory perception and dowsing—better known as water divining—topics that, apart from healing, were quite new to me.

I had never been interested in the so-called paranormal— nor, for that matter, in science fiction, mystery stories, or romance novels. Fact, not fiction engaged me; tales of men and women who overcome some adversity in life. Yet I also relished a new experience, so when a friend invited me to the seminar, I readily accepted.

Bruce told us he discovered his healing gift while serving in France during the Second World War. Finding himself with a severely wounded comrade and no medical assistance in the field, he felt impelled to place his hand on the soldier's open wound. To his surprise, the young man's pain quickly abated, as did the effects of shock.

"This happened again," said Bruce, "too often to have been mere coincidence. As a result of these experiences, I decided to devote my life to healing after the war."

By the time I met him in the 1970s, Bruce was teaching and training healers at his home in Scotland. Seated before him now—hoping he could help me as he had helped others—I tried to silence the skeptical part of my mind and surrender to the trust that came so easily when I was a child.

"Well, now, Faye," he said, removing a pendulum from his pocket and letting it swing between us in a neutral oscillation, "what seems to be the problem?"

The pendulum was Bruce's only diagnostic tool. According to the *yes* or *no* question he asked mentally, the direction of its swing gave him the answer. I watched the bob move to and fro, wondering how to frame my reply. There were so many problems I hardly knew where to begin.

"Well, Bruce, for a start I can't sleep. I keep waking at two in the morning with a grinding headache, my joints are stiffening and my hair is falling out. I feel exhausted much of the time, which isn't like me at all, and I think I'm going mad. Shall I go on?"

"Hmmm." The pendulum began to turn in a clockwise direction. "Have you had your flat checked for noxious energies?" he asked.

"No. Why?"

"I think you may have a black stream running through it." The spin grew stronger. "If I were you, I would find a good dowser to check this out. I'd be glad to do it for you, but I'm returning to Scotland tomorrow."

I knew from Bruce's seminars that "black streams" and "noxious energy fields" are terms dowsers use to describe earth's fractured energy lines. These are invisible lines that rise like walls of energy from deep within the earth—how high we do not know—but they appear to be part of earth's planetary design. Benign in their normal, nature-created pattern, when the lines become fractured or cross through a polluted stream, their effect on sensitive people, if exposed to them for any length of time, can be malefic.

I promised Bruce I would get a dowser to vet the flat as soon as possible, although I found it hard to believe that something as nebulous as an invisible energy line could be the cause of my very tangible symptoms. Bruce turned his attention then to my spine, resting his hands on my lower back for several minutes, before consigning me to one of his trainee healers, who now did most of the work.

Seating me on the massage table, she rested her hands gently on my back above the shoulder blades. A lovely warmth began to spread through my being. I thought of the many healers to whom I had submitted my hapless body over the years, each time hoping that this person or that therapy would be the one to effect the longed-for miracle. Yet, dedicated though each practitioner was, I think I knew that whatever was wrong with me, it would not be cured by a simple laying-on of hands.

As soon as I reached home, I rang a friend who was collaborating with a well-known writer on an anthology of the paranormal. The term covers a broad range of phenomena, of which dowsing is mistakenly thought to be one. Dowsers regard the gift as a sense we all once possessed, but which has fallen into disuse as the distractions of civilization draw us away from our at-one-ment with the environment.

"Ruth," I said, "would you know of a dowser who specializes in earth energies? I think I may have a black stream going through my flat."

"I do, actually," she replied. "There's a retired wing commander in Maidenhead who is an expert on noxious energies. His name is Clive Beadon and he is a former president of the British Dowsing Society. You can probably get his phone number through the Maidenhead exchange."

I reached Clive Beadon at his home the next day.

"I'm afraid I can't help you at the moment," said the odd, high-pitched voice on the telephone. "I'm leaving for Arizona tomorrow to find water in the desert for an American company. I'll be gone for about ten days, but if you can send me a map of your property, I'll have a look at the problem when I get back and ring you as soon as I can check things out on site."

Clive Beadon's request for a map on which to determine if an invisible energy line went through my flat was not as daft as it might appear; Bruce's seminars also covered the phenomenon of map dowsing. Improbable though it may seem, any skilled dowser wishing to locate a source of water, or oil, or a hidden pipe, or any other object buried on a property, however distant, can find it as easily on a map of the area, using a pendulum, as on the property itself, assuming it is there. Why this should be, not even dowsers can explain. That it works is proved when water is found on the site within a foot of where the dowser located it on a map and he collects his fee.

The idea that a mere representation of a property miles away can yield information about that property beggars belief. The implications for our Euclidian concepts of image

16

and space are mind-boggling. A map dowser works with the paradox that things have not only to be seen to be believed, they must be believed to be seen.

In 1933, Alfred Korzybski wrote, in *Science and Sanity,* "The map is not the territory." Korzybski, it appears, was wrong. In the strange world of dowsing, the map *is* the territory.

CHAPTER FOUR

Magic is the term we use for the mysterious
and the inexplicable.
—Graham Green

Wing commander Clive Beadon, DFC, was the very model of a 1940s Royal Air Force officer. Tall, late sixties, with ginger brows bristling above blue eyes, he was wearing fawn trousers and a brown blazer, the RAF buttons gleaming like bright little badges of authority. Only after his death did I learn of the wartime exploit for which he was awarded the Distinguished Flying Cross.

> In 1944, Clive Beadon flew a Liberator bomber at low level to attack Japanese supply trains on the Bangkok-Chiengmai railway. His aircraft was hit by Japanese anti-aircraft fire, its tail destroyed, its gunner killed and the rear portion set ablaze. Beadon struggled to maintain height and somehow succeeded in piloting the burning Liberator more than 1,000 miles back to base.[1]

He was standing as if at attention when I opened the door, a briefcase in one hand, a wooden box tucked under the other arm. Faintly awed, I invited him in and we exchanged

---

[1] Excerpt from Clive Beadon's obituary in the *Daily Telegraph,* September 16, 1996.

civilities in the entrance hall. He placed his briefcase and box on the hall table, before turning to address me in those clipped pukka vowels I had heard on the telephone:

"Now then, I'd like to show you what I found on your map."

He snapped open the case and removed the blueprint I'd sent him of the flat. Spreading it out on the table he explained, "I've marked only the major lines here, but there are many more." I peered at the map, now so crisscrossed with lines it looked as though someone had scattered chopsticks all over the rooms. "As you can see," said Beadon, "it's a very disturbed situation you have here. In fact, I haven't seen so many lines going through a property before."

"What do they mean?" I asked anxiously, raising my eyes from the map.

"We'll discuss that in a moment," he said. "But first, I would like to do a quick dowse of the flat, if I may."

He turned again to his briefcase and withdrew a whalebone divining rod—also called the Y-rod because of its shape, the contemporary version of the forked twig still used by some country dowsers. Next, he opened the wooden box to reveal a warren of compartments filled with curious objects: polished gemstones of various colors and shapes, small vials containing mysterious liquids, several pendulums, and a plastic disk three inches in diameter that was divided into different colored segments.

Selecting the disk, Beadon palmed it in one hand before grasping both ends of the rod and setting it in the horizontal "search" position. He then paused for a moment and lifted his head, as though harking to something. Placing his ring finger on one segment of the disk, he stepped toward the corridor, saying, as though to himself, "Now there should be a red line . . . about here." At the word "here," the rod rose to a perpendicular position.[2] Beadon brought both ends of the

---

[2] For most dowsers in the British Isles, the Y-rod points up to indicate "yes," whereas in the U.S., it usually points down. We don't know why.

rod together to break the hold, then took several steps into the corridor, murmuring, "And another line . . . about here." Again the rod rose, as if on cue.

Beguiled by the thought of invisible lines that respond to color, I followed him as he walked through the rooms, the rod rising and falling as he went. I longed to ask what the disk was for but didn't for fear of putting him off his stride. Besides, he was just the teeniest bit intimidating.

At the end of the dowse, we were in the sitting room. Beadon closed the rod and placed it with the disk on the coffee table.

"Now then," he said, "as I observed before, it's a very disturbed situation you have here. Frankly, I'm not surprised you've had so many health problems."

"Do sit down and tell me what you've found," I said, eagerly.

Beadon eased himself into the sofa and leaned back against the cushion.

"For a start," he said, threading his fingers across his chest, "you have a polluted stream running diagonally under your bed, about seventy-five feet down. You also have five energy lines that cross through the bed where your chest would be when you sleep. Some of these lines also traverse the stream, which can't have been doing you much good either. When these energies cross a polluted stream, their negative influence is increased."

"Then you think *they* could be causing my symptoms?" I said, trying not to look as skeptical as I felt.

"I'm almost sure of it," he said, with a confident smile.

"It's hard to believe my headaches and stiffening joints could be caused by something as nebulous as sleeping over a polluted stream or in crossed energy lines," I confessed.

"Not 'caused,'" Beadon corrected me. "They merely exacerbate a latent tendency for those conditions. You see, geopathic radiation, which is what this is called, disrupts the metabolism—of plants as well as people—and can weaken the immune system. Unfortunately," he added, "the average person is not aware of this—nor, for that matter, is the

20

average doctor. Of course," he sniffed, "the medical profession keeps saying it needs more than anecdotal evidence before this can be accepted, yet when proof is offered, it is dismissed out of hand."

"Well, you must admit," I said, trying not to smile, "that terms such as 'black streams' and 'invisible energy lines' do invite a certain skepticism."

"Of course they do," he conceded. "Nonetheless, everything in nature identifies itself by color, even if the color is invisible. Now this disk," he said, reaching for it on the coffee table, "is divided into eight colors—or six, if you discount the black and white sections. It's called the 'Mager Rosette,' after the Frenchman who invented it, but I call it the 'color wheel.' When searching for water, if you hold the wheel in your hand thusly, with your finger touching the blue or white segment, your rod will respond only to pure water. Brackish or polluted water responds to grey or black, which may be where the term 'black stream' comes from."

"I had no idea dowsing could be so complicated," I said. "I've done a few experiments with the pendulum, but I still don't understand how it works."

"Neither do I," said Beadon, cheerfully, "it just does. And frankly, I'm not much interested in theory. Success in dowsing is based on intent and visualization. If one's intent is focused, the unconscious kicks in and one's dowsing becomes more accurate.

"For example," he explained, "to find a vein of water you must think deep into the earth and visualize a running stream. It can be a quite narrow one, but it should be flowing through granite rock. Oddly enough, still water, such as a lake or a pond, doesn't emit these radiations. The reason it helps to use color when trying to distinguish a stream from an energy line, is because the latter are picked up on red or yellow.

"Now, your problem," he added, "appears to be that you react unconsciously to these energies, which is why you have been troubled by the stream under your bed and the crossed lines. So you'll need to learn how to control your sensitivity."

He paused, looked at me for a moment, then said, as though an idea had just occurred to him, "I say . . . given your sensitivity to these lines, I might use you as a guinea pig for the control I'm working on."

"Oh? What kind of control?" I asked, my interest quickening.

"To shield people from the harmful effects of geopathic stress, which is what these energies cause when they become fractured. I've been trying to find a better way of neutralizing them than the methods that hitherto have been applied, which is why I developed the spiral."

"The spiral?"

"The name I've given the control I'm working on—'The spiral of tranquility.' However," he added, glancing at his watch, "I'm afraid I haven't time to go into that now; I have an appointment in Maida Vale at four."

The twinge of regret I felt at his leaving surprised me. It was a long time since a subject held me so enthralled. As we walked to the entrance hall, I said,

"I do hope you can do something about these wretched energies, whatever they are."

"I'll do my best," said Beadon, with the sort of smile that did not countenance failure. "Now, I'll try to have a control ready for you in a week or so. In the meantime, if you would like to practice finding the stream in your bedroom, I can leave my rod and color wheel here for you to play with. Oh, don't worry," he added, staying the protest he saw on my lips, "I always carry an extra set with me."

He closed the wooden box, snapped his briefcase shut and swept both off the table.

"Well, good-bye, my dear," he said at the door and stepped onto the landing to press the bell for the lift. Six floors down, its ancient mechanism cranked noisily into gear for the slow, rickety ascent to the top. Too impatient to wait, Beadon started down the stairs, his balding head disappearing behind the lift shaft as he waved good-bye.

I closed the door and stood in the hall for a moment, thinking of the strange new world that had just opened up to me. It was as though I had been shown an alternate reality in which water, my friend since childhood, could become an enemy when polluted, even if I didn't know it was there. How I envied dowsers who could shut down their sensitivity when it wasn't needed—who had to *search* for a polluted stream, instead of try to avoid its radiations.

Freed from Beadon's intimidating presence, I decided to see if I could find the stream in my bedroom, using his rod and the wheel. Holding them in the same way he did, I stood at the head of the bed and placed my ring finger on the black segment of the disc. Walking slowly forward, I tried to visualize a narrow stream running through walls of granite rock deep in the earth. When I neared the corner, the rod began to rise, as though an unseen hand was pushing it up from below. I turned to traverse the foot of the bed and the rod relaxed, returning to the horizontal search position. I continued to walk up the other side of the bed. When I neared the headboard, the rod rose again—confirming the stream's diagonal path, as Beadon described.

But was the force I felt pushing against the rod really the radiation from an underground stream? Or had I created it subconsciously, because of Beadon's suggestion?

As I pondered the interaction of image, energy and thought, it occurred to me that if we can find a polluted stream simply by thinking deep into the earth, what might we discover by thinking high into the heavens—by tuning in to the infinite, so to speak, or to universal mind or cosmic consciousness or God or whatever we want to call it?

CHAPTER FIVE

I thank God for all those genial hours in which
He has allowed me to forget Him.
—Philip Toynbee

In the weeks following Clive Beadon's visit, my symptoms grew rapidly worse. When I walked in the park the earth rejected me with its mold and the grass with its pollen. While I slept, the stream's radiations invaded my body, stiffening my joints and draining my strength. How could I live in a world where even nature turned against me? Only the flowers lifted their friendly faces toward me, yet even some of these—the loveliest and most fragrant—sickened me with their scent.

My body had become a human pendulum, reacting, it seemed, to every shift in the environment. Even my heart abandoned its normal rhythm, skipping beats one moment and speeding up the next. In Harrods one day I nearly fainted when it began to flutter like a trapped pigeon, stopped suddenly, and then resumed its thumping with slow heavy thuds against my chest. Days later, an electrocardiogram showed my heart to be perfectly sound.

It was mid-June when Beadon delivered his Spiral of Tranquility, which I hoped would neutralize the energies he claimed were affecting me in my flat.

"Sorry I couldn't get this to you sooner," he said, removing a small box from his briefcase and handing it to me. "My wife has been ill—she has a bad heart—and the jobs have been piling up. I'm afraid I can't stay long," he added, waving aside my offer of a drink.

I opened the box to find an acrylic block two inches square, with a copper spiral in the center surrounded by floating gemstone chips. Entranced with its oddity I asked,

"What are the gemstones for?"

"Well, dowsers have known for ages that copper can divert some of these broken energy lines from a property, but I found that copper alone doesn't do the job. This troubled me, so I looked for a method that would take care of the rest."

"What led you to try gemstones?"

"I don't know why it occurred to me to experiment with crystals, but I found that certain stones, if placed at the point of entry on a map of the property, will block these lines without sending the problem on to someone else. One must take great care when attempting to change the environment. By adding the correct stones to the copper, the control seemed to achieve better staying power."

"I see," I lied, not seeing at all how crystals and copper could thwart a determined energy line.

"Now I'm going to leave this control with you," he said. "As long as you keep it in the open on a wooden surface— not glass, glass will fracture the lines—it should deflect both the energy lines and the influence of the stream. I'll ring you in a few days and you can tell me if things have calmed down."

The flat did feel more tranquil for a day or two, but then the telltale symptoms crept back. When Beadon rang for his report, I had to deliver the disappointing news.

"How tiresome," he said, meditatively. "I shall have to rethink the situation in your flat."

The same thing happened with his next spiral and with the one after that—palpable relief for forty-eight hours, only to feel the symptoms slowly return. Once, a sudden compression in my lungs made me wonder if a stone in Clive's latest control could be the cause, for I seemed to be peculiarly sensitive to his crystals. When the pressure increased, I grew alarmed and rang him in Maidenhead.

"Absolutely not," he replied. "If you were going to be bothered by one of the stones, you would have felt it before now." But then he glanced at the maps spread out in his study and saw that he had left a malachite stone lying on a corner of mine. When he removed the stone, within moments the pressure eased, to our surprise.

"You're a very queer fish, aren't you," said Clive, with a touch of annoyance in his voice.

Another time, he inadvertently placed a small mirror on my map, which crossed one of the energy lines, thus splitting it in two. This prompted another emergency call to Maidenhead. Apparently, the line the mirror fractured on my map fractured the one in my flat as well, creating a discomfort that vanished as soon as the mirror was removed.

The third time this happened, Clive said,

"I say . . . there's something I would like to try. Do you have your pendulum handy? Good. Now, don't hang up. Go stand in one of those energy lines by your bed, pick up the phone there and let me know what the pendulum's doing."

I did as he instructed, positioning myself by the telephone at the head of the bed.

"I'm standing over the stream now," I reported, "or perhaps it's a line. I'm not sure which."

"Doesn't matter. Pendulum going around? Fine. Now I'm going to do something to your map here and I want you to tell me if the pendulum changes its swing in any way."

I wondered what Beadon could be doing as I watched the bob swing vigorously in a clockwise circle, then begin to decelerate.

"It's slowing down, Clive," I reported. "Wait . . . now it's still. What have you done?"

"Never mind. Just tell me if it starts up again."

It did, moments later. This game—for that's what it seemed to me at the time—continued for twenty minutes or so, the pendulum spinning in one direction, slowing down, then reversing its spin or adopting a diagonal swing—all in response to something Beadon was doing, apparently, to a map of my flat miles away. There was no question of my influencing the pendulum's movements for I had no idea what he was up to—or why.

Eventually, he said, "I may have found the stones that will take care of your problem. I'll make a mock-up control and bring it round when I'm next in London."

This was the first of what would become six years of long-distance dowsing experiments over the telephone. Each time a test spiral broke down, Clive returned to the dowsing board, puzzled but unbowed. As a result of these failures I became his guinea pig, though in ways that neither of us could have imagined.

On one visit he complained, only half-jokingly: "I can't understand why you're such a problem; none of my other clients give me such a hard time."

"That's because I'm not a client anymore," I retorted. "I'm a guinea pig and I'm having a hard time with your guinea piggery."

Clive shot me a rueful glance. "Well, if I can block you, I can block anyone."

Much as he relished a challenge, Clive was finding the problems in my flat more vexatious than he'd anticipated. As the months wore on and one disappointment followed another, the stress began to tell on us both. For Clive, it meant more work for me when he had important jobs to do and dowsing seminars to prepare. For me, it meant an ever-deepening discouragement.

One day in September, after another spiral broke down, he said, "You know, given the pernicious nature of these energies, you might want to think about moving."

"Moving!" I exclaimed, the mere thought so disheartening I refused even to consider it. *"I will not run away from this problem!"* I wrote in my diary that night, with the sense of having written my epitaph. Meanwhile, I was growing more feeble by the day and no one could tell me why.

In October, calluses began to form on the soles of my feet, sores appeared on the roof of my mouth and rashes broke out on different areas of my body. At night, I woke with an inchoate fear and the sense that my sanity was slipping away. What on earth was happening to me? If only I knew. If only someone knew. By December, I was tempted to abandon the book on adoption and write about this experience instead. But a book about an illness with no name, no known cause, and no cure at the end? Hard enough to live; impossible to read.

My daughter, Amy, had applied for admission to a college in New York, so on the 17th we flew to that city to do a tour of inspection. While there, my symptoms abated to some extent, lending credence to Clive's conviction that the problem lay primarily in my flat. At a dinner party the night before our departure, I indulged in my three worst addictions: chocolate, coffee and cheese. My stomach had always accommodated whatever I fed it, but that night, as my fingers turned red and began to throb, I knew that food must have something to do with my condition.

Proof came the next morning, when I woke feeling as though a steel rod had been rammed through my skull. I had no painkillers, so by the time we reached the airport I was in agony. Flying often brought on a headache, but this was the first time I embarked with one. No alcoholic hangover could rival the pain that kept pounding in my skull throughout the long flight back to London.

By March 1983, the calluses on the soles of my feet had thickened and spread to the heels. When my right foot developed a lingering pain, I made an appointment to see the woman doctor I had avoided since our first meeting. She happened to be away, so I saw her locum[3] instead—a breezy young man who was seeing patients as though sizing eggs on a conveyor belt.

"But what should I do if my foot gets worse over the long Easter weekend?" I asked, when he dismissed the pain as insignificant.

---

[3] Deputy acting for a doctor.

"Well, it will just be Murphy's Law then, won't it?" he said, cheerfully.

"Murphy's Law?"

"If things can possibly get worse at the worst possible time, they will."

"That's not very reassuring," I said.

"That's life," he shrugged.

That's the caring NHS.

Days later, an X-ray failed to show any cause for the pain in my foot. Gazing at its skeleton on the screen, however, I was reminded of when I was eight or nine and my mother took me to Bullocks Wilshire to buy my clothes. The children's shoe department had a wondrous toy—an X-ray machine! If I slid my feet into the space at the bottom and looked down through a window, I could see the bones in my toes and watch them wiggle inside the shoes. I cringe now to think of the minutes I spent playing this innocent game. How many roentgens were absorbed by young bones in the 1930s before the danger of those machines was realized and they were removed? How many adult cancers could be traced to those lingering childhood exposures?

By mid-April, the soles of my feet were so sensitive I could hardly bear to wear normal shoes. Going barefoot at home, I kept stubbing my toes and managed to break one on my right foot. When, oh, *when* would I ever walk again without pain?

The energy lines, too, seemed to be growing stronger. There were nights when I couldn't stay in the flat and had to doss down with a sleeping bag in the home of an indulgent friend, only to find that her environment was almost as disturbed as my own. Why, then, didn't *she* feel these energies, too?

How strange I must have seemed to my friends at this time; how strange I seem to myself now, after all these years. My distress, however, was not imaginary. It was as real as if someone had strung an electrical wire through my body and turned the alternating current on "high."

When yet another control broke down, I began to reconsider Clive's suggestion that I move. After all, I reasoned, to move does not necessarily mean to run away; it could even mean to go forward. Having thus rationalized my compliance, in April of 1983, I began to look for another flat.

I found one in an old building that was being renovated on Onslow Square. Before committing to it, however, I asked the estate agent if I could have a friend look it over. Accordingly, on the appointed day Clive joined us at number Seven and did a walk-through dowse of the rooms. Trotting along behind him with my own color wheel and rod, at one point I caught sight of the agent's face; it seemed to be saying, "Crikey! I've got a couple of right Charlies here!"

At the end of the dowse, Clive folded his rod and said, "Well, the bedroom is clear. I can find nothing here that should disturb you."

With this assurance, I took the flat and booked the move for the 7th of June, wondering how I was going to manage all the packing in my debilitated state. Amy was still at school and Kate had left home to live with a boyfriend. To avoid imposing further on friends, with Tony's help I moved Kate's mattress into the empty flat and slept on the floor until the furniture arrived. It did feel a bit spooky at night, since I was the only one in the building and I had no telephone.

With the move only a month away, the demands on my diminishing strength increased. On the 8th of May, wall-to-wall carpeting was installed in the flat. That night, I thought I was going to die. Stricken with a mysterious illness I lay in the dark, reflecting that if I died I would die without knowing what had taken my life. For two days I was bed-ridden with bone-aching fatigue, a hammering head, and a heart that threatened to pack up altogether. Why did my brain keep insisting that I was basically sound, when my body kept screaming that I was falling apart? For fifty years I had viewed the sick from the vantage of health. Now, I gazed at the healthy with the envy of illness.

By the end of the week, I had almost recovered, but then I tripped over some tools left by a carpenter in the hallway and broke another toe. How on earth was I going to cope with the move in three weeks' time?

The move to Onslow Square was a triumph of necessity over infirmity, which sent me back to bed for another two days. The calluses on my feet developed fissures that started to bleed, and by the end of the month a dark crust had formed over the weeping soles. It was like having the stigmata while lacking the strong religious faith that would have given it meaning.

Unfortunately, I had recently attended a private screening of a documentary about a young man who was afflicted with ichthyosis. This is a hideous disease that causes the surface of the skin to become rough and scaly, like the scales on a fish. The man's back and arms, black from the dirt collected in the crevices, bore an alarming resemblance to the scales on my feet.

The film recorded the attempt of a hypnotherapist to arrest the progress of the disease through hypnotic suggestion. Remarkably, he succeeded in restoring some of the man's epidermis to its normal state. But then a doctor informed him that ichthyosis is congenital, and therefore incurable. From that moment on, the hypnotist lost his power to influence the condition.

The fact that ichthyosis is hereditary should have fore-stalled the morbid fears that were forming in my mind, for I knew enough of the medical history of both my birth parents by then to dispel such fevered imaginings. At the time, however, I wondered if the crusts accreting on the soles of my feet—like barnacles on the hull of a ship—could be hereditary, and thus the first stage of this disfiguring and appalling disease.

CHAPTER SIX

Despise no new accident in your body,
But ask opinion of it.
—Bacon

In September, I learned of a Dr. Choy at the Humana Wellington Hospital who was studying the effect of electricity on sensitive people. I spoke with him on the phone and he suggested I see his colleague, Dr. Monro.

"She's very interested in problems like yours," he said. "I can give you an appointment for the 20th."

When I arrived at Dr. Monro's office, the receptionist handed me the customary *New Patient Questionnaire*. This one, however, was unlike any I had seen before. In addition to the usual questions about symptoms and past operations, it asked about my home environment: What sort of cleaning products did I use? What type of cooking and heating fuel—gas or electricity? Were carpets, curtains and furniture coverings made of cotton or synthetic fibers? Simply by having to think about these things for the first time, I became aware of them in a way that hadn't occurred to me before.

Dr. Monro also came as a surprise. Young and attractive, with honey-colored hair swept into a twist, her manner was sympathetic and her voice as soft as that of a young girl. Beneath her gentle exterior, however, Jean Monro had a spine of tempered steel. She needed one, for pitted against her was the British medical establishment—as hostile to the unorthodox in England as the American Medical Association (AMA) is in this country.

Dr. Monro studied my questionnaire for several minutes, glancing up to inquire about a particular symptom, as though it was significant instead of imaginary.

"I hope you don't think my symptoms too weird," I said.

"Not at all," she replied with a smile. "We're quite open-minded about things here." Dr. Monro thought my problems could be caused by allergy and suggested I have some testing done to determine my "frequencies"—whatever those were. "For the moment, the testing procedure is being done at my home in Kings Langley," she explained, "while we complete negotiations for space in another hospital in London."

She scheduled my appointment and gave me directions to her home. I left her office with a feeling of renewed, if cautious hope. I liked Jean Monro. She had none of the self-importance of some of her male colleagues. Even if her treatment should fail, I reflected, it will be an interesting learning experience.

I arrived at her home in Hertfordshire on the 7th of October, only to be brought up short by a notice on the front door:

IF YOU ARE WEARING PERFUME, COLOGNE, OR HAIRSPRAY, OR IF YOU SMELL OF TOBACCO SMOKE, PLEASE DO NOT ENTER. RING FOR THE NURSE.

No one had warned me. The touch of cologne I dabbed on my wrist that morning was an absent-minded concession to a habit I had all but abandoned. The thought of having come all that way, only to find I could not be tested, sent my spirits plummeting. I rang the bell. A nurse came to the door. I explained my predicament and she went to fetch Dr. Monro.

"I'm so sorry," said Dr. Monro. "You should have been given these instructions in advance. We have some very sick people here who are highly sensitive to chemicals. If you don't mind washing off your perfume with soap in the upstairs bathroom you can stay. You'll find a cotton shirt hanging on a hook there, which you can put on afterwards, because some of the scent could still cling to your blouse."

I went upstairs and scrubbed the offending cologne from my skin, keeping a watchful eye on the large spider poised at the edge of the sink. After donning the shirt I returned downstairs, but before I could enter the testing room I had to pass a "sniff" test by the nurse, to ensure that no scent remained on my skin.

There was only one patient in the room—a young woman in her thirties whose feet were severely deformed with arthritis. I tried not to think what mine would be like if the calluses grew much worse. The cracks on my heels were so painful the only shoes I could tolerate now were sandals, yet even in these I walked with the tread of a leper.

The nurse returned with some long narrow boxes labeled "wheat," "corn," "molds," "house dust mite," "monosodium glutamate" and so forth.

"These are antigens," she explained. "An antigen is a substance capable of stimulating an immune response. Each box contains ten vials filled with homeopathic doses of a single antigen suspended in a saline solution. Homeopathy is a system of treating diseases with minute doses of a natural substance which, in healthy people, would produce symptoms similar to the disease. Of course, all the foods used in these antigens are organically grown."

"How does the treatment work?" I asked, intrigued.

"The vials are numbered 1 to 10. The higher the number the weaker the antigen. The testing procedure, called 'skin titration,' involves injecting a dose of the antigen into the skin of the upper arm in serial dilutions. These intradermal injections produce a raised wheal and we always start with wheat #2, because wheat is one of the most common allergens."

She injected wheat #2 into my arm and a wheal quickly appeared. Removing a small ruler from her breast pocket, the nurse measured its size and set the timer on the table for ten minutes.

"When the timer rings, I'll measure the wheal again. If it has grown, you're deemed sensitive to the substance and a weaker dilution, #3, will be injected. We continue this procedure until the neutralizing dose—or 'end point'—is reached. That's the amount that does not provoke a symptom or increase the size of the wheal."

"And the neutralizing dose stops the reaction?"

"It neutralizes reactions to foods, pollens, chemicals, and any other substances the body regards as hostile. This allows it to build up its immune system so that future encounters with these substances can be tolerated. Of course as the patient improves the end point changes, so retesting is periodically required."

While she was speaking, Dr. Monro entered the room and continued the explanation.

"Patients are rarely sensitive to just one group of antigens," she said. "In some patients, reactions will occur chiefly to chemicals, while in others it will be to foods or inhaled particles. However," she cautioned, "the desensitizing drops act slowly and only if allergenic foods are eaten in moderation. The drops do not protect against bingeing, nor do they cure addiction. They control symptoms."

I was to record the antigen number and any symptoms that occurred during the ten-minute interval. There were none with the first dose, but when the timer rang the wheal had grown, so the nurse injected wheat #3 into my arm. Within minutes my legs grew stiff, my hands turned crimson and an uncomfortable wave of heat went through my body. This continued until we reached my end point of #7.

Noting my scarlet fingers, the nurse took hold of my hands and turned them over to inspect the palms. "You certainly are allergic to wheat, aren't you?" she said.

"I'm certainly addicted to it," I confessed, "but how can I be allergic to something I eat every day?"

"That's called 'masked allergy,'" she explained. "It masks as an addiction. Withdrawal from the food produces the same sort of craving the smoker has when deprived of a cigarette. The body struggles to adapt to the allergen by producing symptoms that have no apparent relation to the substance itself, and because we are all different each patient may react differently to the same substance."

The concept of allergy as addiction was new to me. If true, it might explain why doctors, who diagnose according to symptoms, can be confused by conditions that fail to conform to a known pathological pattern. After all, they can't diagnose what they don't know exists.

"At the end of the session," the nurse continued, "your end-point dose will be placed in a dropper bottle to be taken sublingually four times a day. For patients with multiple allergies, ten antigens can be combined in a single vacutainer for self-injection."

It soon became apparent that testing could be a time-consuming business, especially if a patient reacted strongly to a substance and required successive injections. By this time, the room was filling up and I fell into conversation with the pretty young woman sitting next to me. Her name was Amanda and I learned that she was one of Dr. Monro's earliest and sickest patients. Her story was so unusual it had been written up in the papers. Many of Dr. Monro's patients first learned of her practice through reading about Amanda.

"When Jean found me two years ago," she said (all Dr. Monro's patients called her "Jean"), "I was a 'universal reactor'—you know, sensitive to everything in the environment—what the papers call 'allergic to the twentieth century.' My hair had fallen out and I was so discouraged I tried to end my life twice.

"Jean put me up in an old trailer here in her backyard, with just a bed and cotton curtains at the windows. I lived in it for a year while she treated me. The trailer had to be old," Amanda explained, "so that all its toxic odors, like formaldehyde, had outgassed. The only clothing I could tolerate against my skin was a cotton shift and the few things I could eat had to be brought to me from the kitchen, because I couldn't touch metal cooking utensils."

It was hard to believe Amanda could have been so ill, for her hair was now long and lustrous and she was able to lead a normal, if careful life. Most of the people in the room that day were leading lives of quiet desperation. It was like discovering I belonged to a club I had no wish to join, but of which I had been an unwitting member for years. Invisibly maimed, we were a fellowship of freaks. Our symptoms may have differed, but the process that brought us together was the same—the long, discouraging search for a cure that kept leading to skeptical doctors and the dead end of psychogenic dismissal. If some of us were allergic to the twentieth century, maybe there was something wrong with the century.

I noticed the nurse occasionally referred to a book that lay on the corner table. I asked her what it was.

"It's called *Allergy: Your Hidden Enemy*, by Dr. Theron Randolph," she said. "Dr. Randolph is the father of clinical ecology. Every doctor and every allergy patient should read this book." I glanced through it and decided to buy a copy at my neighborhood Waterstone's on the way home.

Settling down with the book after dinner, I read no further than the dedication when I knew that its author was the kind of doctor I had been seeking for years.

> This book is dedicated to all patients who have ever been called neurotic, hypochondriac, hysterical, or starved for attention, while actually suffering from environmentally induced illness.

At last! Someone who understood. Someone who risked the scorn of his colleagues to help the patients they had abandoned. Hungrily, I read about hidden addiction, the chemicals in our food, the pollution in our air, the poisons in our water, and the price we are paying for our reckless disregard of nature. I discovered that the questionnaire I filled in for Dr. Monro was the one Randolph devised for his patients in Chicago. I learned that many hyper-allergic people grow sicker gradually over a period of years through small, incremental exposures to environmental toxins.

> Sometimes, however, a pre-existing condition is suddenly made much worse by a massive exposure to an allergy-causing substance.

What could my pre-existing condition have been? I wondered. A fragile immune system? When I met my birth mother in 1977, I learned that she suffered from the same hay fever she passed on to me. As for the "massive exposure to an allergy-causing substance," that could have been the fumes from my father's cigars, which made me a passive smoker for my first nineteen years of life.[4]

I thought of the friend who said, "Isn't it odd, Faye, that you lead such a healthy life—I mean, you eat all the right things, you don't drink or smoke or do drugs, yet you have such peculiar physical problems."

It was mortifyingly true. A fish-loving herbivore, I lived on vegetables, fruits, and nuts, ate only whole-meal bread, drank only bottled spring water and decaffeinated coffee (later, a coffee substitute), and took all the prescribed vitamins, minerals, and herbs. Yet my maladies increased, while friends who drank, smoked, and ate the most appalling junk food seemed to thrive—except that two later died of colon cancer in their fifties.

What I didn't know was that plastic bottles leach their plasticizers into the spring water; that the caffeine-removing process left traces of methyl chloride in the coffee; that my coffee substitute was composed of grains, to which I was allergic, and that the binding material of most over-the-counter vitamin pills is wheat or corn—grains again.

---

[4] One cigar contains as many cancer-causing chemicals as a pack of cigarettes. Even if the smoker doesn't inhale, the second-hand smoke causes the same damage.

Worse, my healthy vegetables and fruits were not all that healthy, for they were sprayed with organophosphates, the most toxic of which, DDT, though banned in the U.S., was still exported to third world countries, who return it to us on their heavily sprayed imported produce.

Allergy is a trickster. How could I be allergic to food when I never had a stomach ache? When I ate shellfish with impunity and had a headache only if I drank two glasses of wine? Now I understood why wheat made me sleepy, why fats gave me flushes, why my "hypoallergenic" soap made me sneeze and why some so-called health foods are not so healthy to eat, especially when based on dairy products, wheat, sugar or corn.

Admittedly, allergy is not a winning complaint. A *Camille* sneezing with hay fever instead of coughing with consumption would not have elicited many tears, apart from those streaming from her own rheumy eyes. And as for her lover, Armand—he'd have had a job sustaining his passion for a heroine wheezing with asthma through blocked bronchial tubes.

How different it was when I had cancer. Then, friends rallied round, all sympathy and solicitude, their concern no doubt informed by a mixture of fear and identification: *This could happen to me!* Cancer is serious. With cancer you can die and death is respected. But no one dies of allergies—do they?

I could only bless the fate that led me to a clinical ecology doctor who, instead of seeing in my symptoms a psychological disorder, recognized the lineaments of environmental illness and a collapsing immune system.

CHAPTER SEVEN

Every man takes the limits of his own field
of vision for the limits of the world.
—Schopenhauer

"Before I sign this," said Dr. Thorne, pen poised over the form on his desk, "I would like to know something about the procedure you wish me to authorize."

It was my first meeting with the new NHS doctor I had been assigned to after moving to Onslow Square. I rarely used the National Health, but his signature was required on the form to authorize Jean's treatment.

Tall, careful, and in his thirties, Dr. Thorne was only marginally less remote than his predecessors. But then, I had come to expect wariness from doctors when they learned I was using alternative methods in addition to theirs.

I started to explain the skin titration procedure, but could tell from the way his jaw began to work that he was not in a receptive frame of mind. Shifting to the subject of symptoms, I tried to describe the feeling of an acid crawling under my scalp and that tide in the head that made me feel I was losing my reason.

"I see," he said, lips pursed. "Are you sure you're not creating your illness unconsciously to gain sympathy or attention at home?"

How does one answer such a question? "Well, of course I am. It works a treat every time!"

"No," I said evenly, "I'm a single parent and there's no one at home whose sympathy I could gain." Indeed, when my daughters were home from school, they were too involved in their teen-age activities to give me much thought, let alone sympathy.

Dr. Thorne reflected a moment before signing the forms with an air of condescension, as though performing a distasteful act. I thanked him for his courtesy and left, reproaching myself for making such a poor job of explaining Jean's treatment.

His suggestion that I could be creating my own illness reminded me of the dermatologist I heard on the radio a few nights before. Referring to "patients who fake their allergies," he accused them of subverting what would otherwise have been "effective treatment"—his, presumably—by "taking drugs, creams, and things they know they shouldn't. Dermatological pathomimicry," he called it—confirming a long-held suspicion that for some doctors, blinding us with buncombe is more important than finding a cure. It was our old friend blame-the-victim again, dressed up in highfalutin medico-speak to explain away failed treatment.

Concerned about the gulf that exists between conventional and alternative medicine, I stopped at a bookstore on the way home and bought a copy of Randolph's book to give to Dr. Thorne. Well, he did say he would like to know something about the procedure. The next day I delivered it to his office with a note, thanking him again and saying that I hoped he would find the subject of interest.

"Have you removed the control from your flat?" Clive demanded on the 17th of October. "I've just checked your property on the map here and it appears to be off."

"I had to put it away, Clive. Something was affecting me last night and I couldn't sleep. I put it in a drawer to see if that made a difference."

"And did it?"

"Not really."

"Then put it back."

41

My flat had few secrets from Clive. He had only to swing a pendulum over my map in Maidenhead to determine if there was a change in my environment in London. Intriguing though this long-distance surveillance could be, I didn't fancy him peering into my bedroom with a pendulum during one of Tony's visits when the girls were away at school.

Returning home from the clinic, I would find a message waiting on the answering machine:

"Just to let you know I've been watching this new control overnight and it looks promising. Over and out." Or, "I think I've found the small problem that's been bothering you. I'll be having a shot at it this morning. Ring you later. Over and out."

Old wing commanders never died. At least this one hadn't given up on me—yet. My body, however, seemed to be doing just that.

In November, Jean's practice moved to the Nightingale Hospital in Lisson Grove. By then, the antigen testing had produced some surprising results.

Three days after the test for avocado, a favorite fruit, the wheals on my arm remained swollen and red, like angry spider bites. With the first injection of lettuce, a daily staple, I felt as spaced out as if I had taken several Valium. The spaciness persisted until I reached the end point of #10. It was my strongest reaction to date, although the weakest attenuation. The nurse wouldn't let me drive home until she had given me the "turn-off remedy"—a combination of baking soda, potassium, and vitamin C in 8 ounces of water, which neutralizes most allergic reactions.

On November 15th, I began testing "the nasties"—the nurses' term for the most frequently found chemicals in the environment: phenol, terpene, formalin, chlorine, ethanol, glycerol, Dacron, polyester, and nylon.

"We're going to start you on Mixed Papers this morning," said the nurse, as she prepared the syringe.

"Why papers?" I asked, rolling up my shirt sleeve.

"Because of the chemicals in ink, newsprint, and all kinds of paper," she explained, injecting Papers #3 into my arm.

"Oh, dear, all the things I work with every day. I suppose they're in typewriter ribbon as well?"

"Of course. Almost everyone who is allergic to foods, pollens, or molds also reacts to chemicals, though not all in the same way."

As if to confirm her statement, when I removed the morning paper from my handbag moments later, the patient seated next to me asked,

"Would you mind putting that away? It's the chemicals in the newsprint," she explained, apologetically. "I'm affected by the smell."

I quickly returned the paper to my bag, wondering why I hadn't realized that newsprint could be a problem, given the gray smudges it left on my fingers each morning. More troubling, for me, were the perfumed ads tucked into certain magazines, for their scent permeated the pages and clung to my fingers long after I disposed of the periodical and washed my hands. The nurse's comment, however, coupled with the patient's reaction, reminded me of a passage I had read recently in *Gluttons for Punishment,* by James Erlichman:

> Humans can be ten times more sensitive than animals to toxic chemicals, and in addition, some humans are ten times more sensitive than others.

One woman was so hypersensitive, her neutralizing dose was off the chart—somewhere in the 200's—an attenuation so weak it amounted to the merest memory of a substance. The only way she could be tested was to place successive drops of an antigen on the back of her hand until she reached the dose that turned off her symptoms.

Watching her do this, I exclaimed, "Why, that's like dowsing!"

"Dowsing?" she echoed. "What's that?"

"What you're doing—reacting to something so subtle it can't be seen or measured, like the trace of a toxin."

"Oh," she said, not very interested. My timer went off then and the nurse came to measure the wheal on my arm. By the time she injected me with Papers #4, the conversation had moved on.

Another woman, whose chemical sensitivities were in the 100s, could not be tested by injection either because she was allergic to the nickel in the needle. Her method was to hold each vial of an antigen in turn until she reached the one that did not provoke a reaction. This meant that the smallest trace of a substance in a glass vial—even if she only held the vial against her skin—had the same effect as if it had been injected intravenously.

"My worst reactions were to chlorine," she said. "It caused terrible headaches and exhaustion, and the feeling of being utterly drained."

I thought of my California childhood, much of which was spent in a chlorinated swimming pool gulping down great mouthfuls of the stuff. When I watched the pool man dump buckets of chlorine into the water (there were no standards as to amounts in the 30s), it didn't occur to me the chemical could be harmful or that it might be damaging my eyes when I swam with them open underwater for hours.

The more I observed the reactions of my fellow patients, the more impressed I was by the similarity between allergy and the dowsing response, with one significant difference: Diviners tune in mentally, deliberately to the thing they wish to find, whereas sensitive people react involuntarily—even unwillingly—to influences of which they may not even be aware. Unlike the dowsing response, the allergic reaction cannot be turned off at will. In both cases, however, the reaction is to something so subtle it can't be measured scientifically or even explained.

When complaining of this sensitivity to a friend one day, she remarked, "Do you know what you remind me of? *The Princess and the Pea.*"

We both laughed at this, for in truth, my predicament was almost as absurd as that of Anderson's hyper-delicate heroine. How could I, in my bed on the sixth floor, feel the radiations from a polluted stream seventy feet under the ground? How could the real princess have been kept awake all night and her delicate skin bruised by a pea hidden under seven mattresses, while the common-blood pretend-princess slept soundly in her bed? What a gullible goose the queen must have been, I thought, to believe the princess's hyperesthesia proved her to be of royal blood, when in fact she was just a girl with a broken-down immune system.

I met many such princesses at the clinic—women who were affected by things far less tangible than a pea. For example, one day in the testing room a patient said, "I smell smoke!" This prompted a worried rush to the window. When no sign of smoke could be seen, we returned to our chairs and the nurse did a sniff test of the room. To my chagrin, the culprit proved to be the Lapsang Suchong tea I had just decanted from a thermos, its smoky aroma having reached the woman seated at the farthest end of the room.

Such exaggerated acuity only adds to the sufferer's sense of isolation. A visible disability at least elicits compassion. No one tells the MS sufferer she has willed herself into a wheelchair to gain sympathy, or the polio victim that his paralysis has been self-induced. Yet the environmentally ill (E.I.) must contend not only with their physical distress, but with the skepticism of friends and the suspicion of doctors that they are not quite right in the head. Small wonder if they are driven to despair—not only by their affliction, but by the blank incomprehension of their fellow men.

The discovery of how inimical to health is the smallest amount of chemicals in the body brought a radical change to my way of life. Standing in the supermarket one day, I realized that on all those tempting shelves there was almost nothing I could safely eat—nothing that did not contain colorings, additives, fillers, or preservatives. The tins were lined with phenol, the drinks were in plastic bottles (another phenol hazard), and every product that was boxed, packaged, or frozen, contained sugar or salt. We cared more for the shelf life of our food than we did for the life span of our bodies. Even the labels could not be trusted, for manufacturers were not compelled to list every ingredient to which only a few people might be allergic. Nothing was safe. For the chemically sensitive, the supermarket was a minefield.

I recalled another dietician I'd heard on the radio who declared, "There is *no* evidence whatsoever that chemicals, colorings, or preservatives in our food do us harm."

No doubt when doomsday arrives and we are all keeling over with toxic overload, the penultimate voice to be heard in the land will be that of an "authority" assuring us there is no immediate danger—followed by that of a doctor or psychiatrist telling us it is all in our minds.

CHAPTER EIGHT

The probability that there are forces at work in
the universe of which we have as yet scarcely
an inkling is not too bizarre to entertain.
—Gordon Rattray Taylor

On the 23rd of November, while testing more of the nasties at the clinic, a fierce pain shot through my arm with the first injection of nylon. My fingers throbbed and my heart thumped so violently I needed the turn-off remedy again.

It was during this session that something happened which I am still at a loss to explain. There were five of us in the small room: four women and a man. I was seated next to the corner table, which held the boxes of chemical antigens we were to test that day. The box of Dacron lay open on top, the ten vials exposed.

Seated cater-corner to the table on my right were a man and a woman. A second woman sat opposite me reading a book, while the two women on my left were engaged in conversation with the nurse. She was the only one on duty that morning, although there should have been two, so the testing procedure was taking even longer than usual.

Impatient with the delay, I wondered if I could dowse for my end point; it would save time and avoid those pesky pricks in the arm. I glanced around the room. The man and woman on my right were engrossed in their books, as was the woman directly opposite. The women on my left were still chatting with the nurse.

I opened my handbag and as furtively as possible withdrew my pendulum. Suspending it from the fingers of my left hand, I rested the palm of my right hand on the glass vials, asking mentally, *What number is my end point for Dacron?* I was counting the bob's rotations when a sharp voice said, "Put that pendulum away at once!"

Startled, I looked up to see the nurse glaring at me as she administered a hurried injection to one of the women. "You must *never* use a pendulum where sensitive patients are being tested," she said, angrily. "I *wondered* why these patients suddenly went into reaction."

To my astonishment both women appeared to be in some distress, for which my innocent dowsing was being blamed.

"But they *couldn't* have been affected by what I was doing," I replied, appalled at the idea. "I wasn't even thinking about them; I was merely trying to find my end point for Dacron. Besides, this pendulum is just a bit of plastic. It has no power of its own."

"You may not think so," retorted the nurse, "but it does. We've had this happen before when someone has used a pendulum near sensitive patients."

"But *I'm* sensitive, too," I protested, "and it hasn't hurt me. I don't see how it could possibly harm anyone else."

"Well, it does," said the woman seated nearest me, who appeared the more affected. "That's why our symptoms flared so suddenly."

"Nonsense," I said, "you weren't even aware of what I was doing."

"That doesn't matter," snapped the nurse, rubbing the woman's arm with an alcohol swab at the site of the turn-off injection.

A heated discussion ensued between the four women (the man tactfully abstaining) about the pendulum's power to create a disturbance simply by its swing—a view I hotly denied.

"It can only respond to the thought and *intent* of the dowser," I insisted, "and as my intent was benign, and my thought focused only on myself, I don't see how it could have affected you or anyone else—for good *or* for ill."

"Oh, but it's a well-known fact that the pendulum creates a magnetic field," chimed in the lady sitting opposite me.

"Rubbish," I said, refusing to dignify that canard by challenging her source. "It can't 'create' anything. It simply registers whatever the subconscious mind is picking up at a given moment. If others imagine themselves to be affected, it must be due to suggestion."

"Not so," protested the lady on my left, pointing out that her back was turned to me at the time, so suggestion didn't enter into it.

"I didn't see what you were doing either," added the nurse, "until the change in these patients alerted me to the fact that something had happened."

To all this I listened in bewildered disbelief. It simply wasn't possible my innocent dowsing could have affected the two women, yet it seemed to have done so. Aghast at the thought of harming anyone, I put the pendulum away and apologized—though for what, I didn't know.

Some time later, Dr. Choy entered the room and came over to my chair.

"I'm afraid I must ask you, please, not to use the pendulum when you're in the hospital," he said, in his polite Chinese manner. "I was with a patient on the floor above when she took a sudden turn for the worse and asked me if someone in the hospital was using a pendulum. I said 'no' because I didn't know you had done so, until I returned to this floor and the nurse told me what happened."

My jaw dropped. How could the swing of a plastic bob have affected anyone—least of all someone on another floor? It wasn't the distance I doubted, for distance means nothing in dowsing; my experiments with Clive had been proving that for three years. But intent *does* matter and my intent had been harmless. Bewildered, I apologized again and buried my head in a book for the rest of the session.

As soon as I reached home, I rang Clive to tell him about the incident.

". . . And so there it is, Clive. What do you make of it?"

"Absolute rubbish!" he snorted. "In all my years of using the pendulum and reading about it, I have never heard of such a thing happening. It's nonsense to think you could have affected anyone other than yourself."

"I know. That's what I told them. Yet it happened."

That evening, while recording the incident in my diary, I became aware of a strong chemical odor in the room. It appeared quite suddenly, the way the scent of perfume sometimes hovered over my desk for a minute or two before fading away. Each time this happened I felt it to be my mother's spirit, for it was a joke of long standing that I disliked the heavy floral perfume she favored. That night, however, the odor resembled paint stripper or nail varnish. Was I going mad, or had my olfactory nerves become so sensitive that life on this planet would soon be intolerable?

Two days later, while discussing the incident with Dr. Monro, she told me of an experience she had a year earlier, which led her to ban the use of a pendulum in her clinic.

"A healer was brought in—with the patient's consent, of course—to measure the level of something in her body with a pendulum. Suddenly, the patient went into a coma and it took me three weeks to nurse her back to health. So you see," she added, "I do know that such things can happen."

In the days that followed I turned the matter over and over in my mind, trying to find a rational explanation. A possible, if tenuous one occurred to me:

Each of us in the room that day shared a co-sensitivity to chemicals, which the testing procedure would have intensified. Conceivably, we might have interacted on some unconscious level. My hand was resting on homeopathic vials of Dacron suspended in a saline solution and water is a known conductor of energy.

Did my permeable immune system allow my hand to absorb the Dacron dilutions and transmit them to the women sitting nearest me, whose immune systems were as porous as mine? At the time my body was full of poisons, to which had

50

just been added the fiery injection of nylon. Perhaps the addition of Dacron produced an aura so toxic it affected the sensitive women who were within its perimeter.

But if this is so, what kind of energy are we dealing with? Why wasn't *I* affected as well? Why weren't the other patients in the room affected? And how do we explain the reaction of the woman on the floor above?

The more I ran the incident through my mind, the more incomprehensible it became. And it remains so to this day.

CHAPTER NINE

The medical establishment will only get off
Its pedestal when we get off our knees.
—John Robbins

Three months into the allergy treatment the pain in my foot was gone and the crusts on my feet were starting to heal. I had not had a sneezing spasm for weeks and my eyes stopped watering after house dust mite was added to the antigens. I was now injecting the vaccines, for there were too many to take sublingually. So subtly had these improvements occurred I was scarcely aware of them, pain's remission being less startling than its onset. Still worrying, however, was my hair, which continued to go limp for long periods before regaining some of its curl.

Contemplating of my reaction to the nylon antigen, I recalled my body's rejection of the silicone implant in 1974. In 1980, with a view to reconstruction, I had the same surgeon insert a piece of silicone in my midriff to see if it produced a reaction. If it did, I would abandon the idea. As it happens it didn't, but something told me not to risk the operation.

Now, however, I wanted the piece removed—assuming it could be found, for although it was small, it was still a foreign substance in my body. My surgeon had since died and the tiny scar had disappeared, so I consulted a Harley Street practitioner about the feasibility of the procedure.

Mr. Naylor, as I shall call him (all surgeons in England are addressed as "Mr."), was tall, slim, impeccably groomed and insufferably condescending. As elegant as the silk foulard in his breast pocket, he was all unctuous courtesy and charm—until he heard the word "allergy."

"Of course, I don't believe in allergies," he said.

"Why would my body have rejected the implant if it wasn't allergic to the silicone?" I asked. It seemed a reasonable question.

"You do realize, dear lady," he said, as though addressing a dim chemistry student, "that silicone is an inert substance; therefore, you cannot possibly be allergic to it."

"Unfortunately, Mr. Naylor, I have learned that one can become allergic to almost anything."

He studied me coolly for a moment, his chin resting on long, elegant fingers. Then, "Have you considered seeing a psychiatrist about this?"

I thought I had become inured to the question, but I could feel the rage rising in my gorge.

"No," I said, biting my tongue.

"Why not? Are you afraid to see one?"

"No, I don't need to see one."

"How do you know you don't need to?"

"Are you implying that if I don't see a psychiatrist it's because I'm afraid to, and if I do, I'm admitting my problem is psychosomatic?"

"How do you know it's not psychosomatic?" he countered.

"How do you know that it is?" I shot back. "Have you seen this condition before?"

"Never."

"Then how do you know it's not allergy?"

He sighed and waved a limp hand—like a judge dismissing a tiresome witness from the stand. There being no useful purpose in prolonging the discussion, I was about to leave, when Mr. Naylor made what I can only describe as an immoral suggestion.

"Of course," he said, "I *could* operate on you—take a bit of silicone from somewhere and pretend that I found it in your body."

That such an idea would even occur to the man left me stunned.

"And why would you do that?" I asked, contempt barely under control.

"Well, it would have the same effect, wouldn't it?" he said.

I did not trust myself to reply; it was all I could do to manage a civil good-bye before I fled from his office. *And these are the men we encourage to play God!* I thought. Clearly, the clinic was testing me for the wrong things. I should have been tested for doctor tolerance, ego tolerance, scientific authority tolerance—but not on an empty stomach!

Driving home, the poem of another allergy sufferer kept running through my head. "Yip" Harburg was the brilliant Hollywood lyricist who wrote the lyrics for *The Wizard of Oz*—and for that anthem of the Great Depression, *Brother, Can You Spare a Dime?*

> I'm really not hypochondriacal,
> Though the fear of a seizure cardiacal
> Makes me jumpy and tense and maniacal
> > With each inhalation of breath.
> I'm really not hypochondriacal.
> > I'm merely allergic to death.

At Christmas, a surge of social activity made a shambles of my dietary resolve, turning the diary that was to record my dreams into a record of my recidivism. Bingeing on refined carbohydrates, I understood why the last indulgence granted the prisoner on death row is not sex, but food. If only gluttony made me ill or gave me spots or put fat on my frame, the goad of vanity might have restrained me. But I could lay waste a box of chocolates and have nothing worse to show for it than a guilty conscience and a sense of self-disgust. *That* was the sickening part of it.

In January 1984, while retesting my antigens at the clinic, I found myself sitting next to a weepy Amanda.

"What's the matter, Amanda?" I asked.

"I'm being tested for cow's milk," she said, snuffling, "and it always makes me feel depressed."

A sympathetic patient sought to console her by relating her own experience.

"You know, Amanda, I suffered from indigestion for thirty-four years and the first day they tested me for milk I found I was highly allergic. So I cut out all dairy products for two days and my indigestion disappeared. I haven't touched dairy since."

"But I don't eat dairy products," Amanda replied.

A retired headmistress, who had been listening to the discussion, offered her story.

"I used to have postprandial depression every morning for years and I didn't know why. When they tested me for honey, I became so overwhelmed with sadness I began to weep. I couldn't believe this healthy food I ate for breakfast each morning could be the cause of my depression. Had one of my girls at school behaved the way I was behaving, I would have told her to snap out of it and pull herself together."

Amanda sniffed and made a little show of pulling herself together.

Throughout this conversation we heard muffled screams coming intermittently from an adjacent room. Now, suddenly, the door opened and a young woman emerged, who I recognized as the delightful patient I sat next to the week before. On seeing me, she colored.

"I hope I wasn't making too much noise in there," she said, with a sheepish grin. "When they test me for wheat I become so crazy they need two nurses to hold me down, so I have to be tested in a separate room."

"Good heavens," I said, "does this happen when you eat bread?"

"Oh no, that's what's so odd. But I do have bad premenstrual tension, which wheat seems to exacerbate."

How interesting, I thought. Could it be that some people, diagnosed as psychotic because of behavioral problems, were suffering instead from a food intolerance? Reflecting on the diverse nature of allergy, I turned to Amanda and asked, "Why do you think some of us are allergic to so many things, Amanda, while others aren't affected by them at all?"

"Don't know," she sniffed. "Guess we're just more sensitive."

"Yes, but *why* are we more sensitive?" I persisted. "What has made us so?"

"Just born that way, I guess," she sighed.

But I was born normal; it was only in my forties I became a freak. Of course, genetics had something to do with it, but I didn't think that could be the whole answer.

Half a century ago, Rachel Carson posed the same question in *Silent Spring:*

> What makes one person allergic to dusts or pollen, sensitive to a poison, or susceptible to an infection whereas another is not, is a medical mystery for which there is at present no explanation. ... Some physicians estimate that a third or more of their patients show signs of some form of sensitivity, and that the number is growing. And unfortunately, sensitivity may suddenly develop in a person previously insensitive. In fact, some medical men believe that intermittent exposures to chemicals may produce just such sensitivity.

In January, I saw Dr. Thorne again to obtain his signature on some new forms. It was our first meeting since my visit in October. He signed the forms with the same air of distaste and returned them to me across his desk.

"Was there anything else you wished to see me about?" he asked.

"No, thank you," I replied. But then, wanting him to know that Jean's treatment was helping, I added, "In fact, I'm feeling much better."

This happy news eliciting no flicker of interest or pleasure, I was about to leave, when I remembered he hadn't mentioned the book I left for him in October.

"Oh, by the way, Dr. Thorne, did you receive the book I dropped off for you after our first appointment?"

"I did."

I waited for him to say more. "Well . . . have you read it?"

"No."

"Oh." I murmured something about knowing how busy he must be, but the tone of that "No" pricked my curiosity. "Do you think you will read it, eventually?"

"I may dip into it—I may not."

"I don't understand," I said, "Why wouldn't you?"

"Because I prefer to study the subject in a more structured way, within the framework of my own discipline," he said.

"I see. It was just that . . . I understand allergy isn't included in the syllabus at medical school—at least not in depth—so I thought you might be interested in knowing something about the clinical ecology approach."[5]

He fixed me with eyes as grey as a Gauleiter's. "I'm not interested in some new experimental therapy," he said.

"But it's not new," I protested. "It has been practiced for fifty years. Anyway, isn't every advance in medicine experimental at first?"

"Yes, well, that doesn't concern me. I take the view that I'm here to help you. You are not here to teach me."

I winced. That was *me* put firmly in my place. But why had he taken my gesture as an affront to his authority? Didn't all good doctors learn from their patients? Jean did.

---

[5] In a 1979 survey of U.S. medical schools, 70% of the responding schools indicated they required no formal instruction in occupational or environmental medicine. Among the 30% that did require such instruction, the median time required was four hours during the four years of medical education. In a repeat survey conducted in 1984, 54% of the schools included such instruction, but the median time required was still four hours. Levy (1985).

Randolph did. What did it matter *where* knowledge comes from, as long as we keep learning?

Perhaps, I thought, my lack of education wasn't such a handicap after all, if it saved me from having a discipline into which things needed to fit. Unprejudiced by knowledge, I was freer to make unorthodox connections. Of course, what I still had to learn was that, for some doctors, saving face was more important than opening the mind.

I thought back to the Sunday morning, weeks before, when the energies piercing through me were so strong I didn't think I could bear them much longer. After an agonizing internal debate, I picked up the phone and called Jean. Only desperation could have made me disturb her at home on a Sunday. But instead of resenting the intrusion, as she had every right to do, her response was immediate:

"Can you get here on your own or shall I send a car for you?"

"I think I can make it," I said.

Twice, on the drive to Kings Langley, I almost passed out and had to pull into a lay-by, where I waited, shaking with fear and praying for the strength to go on. When I finally reached Jean's home, she was at the door.

She led me into her kitchen, gave me the turn-off remedy and took my vital signs, while I sat there feeling miserable— and guilty for intruding on her one day of rest. When Jean felt she could leave me, she went to the sitting room and called Dr. Choy.

"Hello, Ray," I heard her say through the open door, "I have Faye here, and . . . ." I forget the conversation, for I was only half-listening, but what I do remember, and what has stayed with me all these years, is the sense of excitement in her voice—as if she were an anthropologist who had just been handed a particularly odd specimen.

"Yes," I heard her say at the end, "isn't it *interesting!*"

Returning to the kitchen, Jean said, "I can't let you drive home in your condition. I think you should spend the night here. You can sleep in the van. It's environmentally safe, and if we cover the windows with aluminum foil, you should be protected from the energies that are affecting you."

Jean fetched some bedclothes from the house, while her son brought a mattress to place on the floor of the van. Then he drove into town to buy some heavy-duty foil to tape over the windows. The foil was useless, of course, as I knew it would be; not even a Faraday cage can block energies that pass through steel.[6]

That night I spent in Jean's van was the longest night of my life. Each minute seemed more unbearable than the last. I thought of Amanda and the year she had lived in Jean's trailer. Did she experience the same physical torment, the same despair, the same fear of losing her mind? But no, this lucid torment was worse than madness. Oh, make me mad, I prayed, so that I may no longer feel! Only the knowledge that I was near the one person who understood—and who cared, even if she couldn't help—enabled me to get through the night.

Recovering my wits in Thorne's office, I said, "We seem to be at cross purposes, Dr. Thorne. In view of the way you feel about the treatment I'm receiving, perhaps you would like me to find another doctor."

"Go right ahead," he said, with withering alacrity.

I left his office feeling more despondent than ever. How could a doctor—a *scientist,* be so uncurious? If *I* had chosen to practice medicine, it would have been for the thrill of discovery; of pushing back the boundaries of knowledge to prove there are *no* incurable diseases, only those for which the cure has yet to be found. I would have searched for that cure, the way an astronomer searches the heavens for a new star—the way Jean was searching—not for honors or wealth or fame, but for a way to help those whom mainstream medicine had abandoned.

---

[6] Michael Faraday, English chemist and physicist, was the inventor of the Faraday cage, a metallic enclosure that prevents the entry or escape of an electromagnetic field.

I drove to the nearest chemist and asked for a list of the NHS doctors in my area. The chemist, at least, was cordial and provided me with their names. Before I could apply to a new GP, however, I received a letter from the Kensington & Chelsea & Westminster Family Practitioner Committee.

Dated February 12, 1984, it ran, "Dr. Thorne has told the Committee that he is no longer willing to be your NHS doctor and has instructed me to remove your name from his list of patients on the 20th of February."

So there it was: The final word, demeaning and official.

That night, as chemical goblins closed in again, I made a solemn pact with the Almighty: *Look, God, you can close as many minds as you like, only please—please close down my sensitivity as well.*

CHAPTER TEN

I would feel more optimistic about a bright future
for man if he spent less time proving that he can
outwit Nature and more time tasting her sweetness
and respecting her seniority.
—E.B. White

In June 1984, Jean learned of a new blood test in America that could identify the presence of any chemical in the body and measure the exact amount, utilizing gas chromatography and mass spectrographic analysis. The technique, developed by a biochemist formerly with NASA, could detect pesticides at levels as low as 0.1 parts per billion.

"This is an important diagnostic advance in the field of clinical ecology," said Jean. "I think we should have you tested for chlorinated pesticides."

"Why pesticides?"

"Because recent studies on patients with possible exposure to the chemical have indicated that levels can remain in the body for as long as twenty years after exposure."

"Twenty years!"

"Yes, one part per billion appears to be the level at which clinical symptoms appear. So the relationship between chemical exposure and clinical symptoms exists at an exceedingly low level. Can you recall any exposures you may have had in the past?"

"Not offhand, no . . . although, when I was on honeymoon in Acapulco, I recall we were having lunch by the pool one day, when a man began spraying the lawn all around the tables. A fine mist fell over our food and I remember thinking, *He must be mad!* But we went on eating, so I guess *we* were the crazy ones.

"Oh, and something else: Each summer, when bugs and spiders crawl into my sitting room from the balcony, I've been killing them with a large insecticide spray gun. I loathe bugs, so I'm sure I spray them much longer than necessary. And then—oh Jean, I'm ashamed to tell you this—I've been closing all the windows and continuing to work at my desk, breathing in those awful fumes for hours. I can't believe now how stupid I've been!"

Jean shook her head at such errant folly, but gave me a forgiving smile. "Well, it's not only insecticides," she said. "It's also organophosphates, which are commonly found in the home. These can cause fatigue, mental confusion, and short-term memory loss, in addition to depression and mood swings."

"All of which I've had, except for the mood swings."

"They can also cause various tingling or pricking sensations, as well as numbness of the limbs."

"But if these things are known, why are such chemicals still being sold?"

"Why indeed," she said. "Anyway, we'll have you tested to see if this could be your problem."

Accordingly, a vacutainer of my blood was drawn and sent to the lab in Louisiana, along with those of some other patients. The results would not be known for several weeks, but Jean felt they could be important in forming a more precise diagnosis.

I had been reading Philip Toynbee's autobiographical *End of a Journey*, written when he was dying of cancer and wrestling with his Roman Catholic faith. Recalling my own struggle with religion in the 1960s, I found his story an absorbing read and closed the book feeling more at peace with my apostasy. *Thank God I'm no longer religious,* I thought—*and thank God I'm not clever enough to be complicated.*

The chemical profiles arrived in July and Jean asked me to come in to discuss mine. I was passing through the glass doors of the hospital, when suddenly, I was reminded of something a medium told me in 1974.

The event that led me to consult a clairvoyant for the first time was finding my original birth certificate while visiting my widowed father in Los Angeles that summer. On discovering my birth parents' names, I was seized by an overpowering desire to find my birth father. His name was Norman Hueston and he would have been seventy by then. Hoping it wasn't too late, I hired a private investigator in Los Angeles to find him for me, because I had to return to England for my daughters' school term.

In London, I confided my search and its urgency to a friend, Ian, who had been trying for several years (unsuccessfully) to interest me in spiritualism. Desperate, now, to find my birth father, I asked Ian if he thought clairvoyance could help me find him more quickly.

"It might," he said, "but only if you go to the very best." He offered to book me a sitting with a medium he knew, but warned me not to be disappointed if nothing came through the first time. "It's not like a tap that can be turned on and off at will, you know," he explained.

Ena Twigg was one of the foremost mediums in England. Such was her fame beyond its shores that letters addressed simply to "Ena Twigg, Medium, England," were delivered to her door. A small woman with dark eyes, black wavy hair and a no-nonsense manner, she might have been any English housewife to whose parlor I had been invited for tea.

I did not tell Mrs. Twigg the reason for my visit, nor did she want to know. At one point, gazing at an invisible screen beyond my right shoulder, she said, "Now I see you going in and out of hotels with glass doors. Not *staying* in them, mind, but going in and out, in and out of glass doors."

This made no sense to me. Why would I be going in and out of hotels, whether I stayed in them or not?

As I passed through the glass doors of the hospital that day, her words came back to me—and it struck me that to a clairvoyant's interpretive eye, the hospital's façade could easily be mistaken for a hotel. Yet why should her words surface in memory only now? At the time, they were forgotten for the next thing she said was so startling, it swept everything else from my mind.

Instead of feeding me dubious messages from my dead adoptive mother, which I was expecting (and was determined to reject), Mrs. Twigg gazed at that invisible screen behind me and said, "Your father is in the other world."

My adoptive father was still alive—so that had to mean Norman was dead. I did not want this to be true.

But then she began waving her hand in front of her face, as though to dispel an unpleasant odor. "Ugh!" she said, "Your father must have been a heavy drinker."

My adoptive father would not allow alcohol in the house.

"I'm afraid you're mistaken," I said. "We are all teetotalers in my family."

"Well, I'm sorry, my dear," she said, holding her ground, *"someone* on your father's side of the family is a heavy drinker, because I'm being *overwhelmed* by the smell of alcohol."

Fear plucked at my solar plexus. She *must* be wrong, I thought. I will find Norman and *prove* her to be wrong!

There was a pause, while Mrs. Twigg appeared to be listening intently to something. Then, very slowly, as though straining to hear each word, she said, "Your father feels remorse for what he did to Sarah."

Sarah was the name of my birth mother, who Norman abandoned when she became pregnant.

"And you have a picture of him, don't you?" added Mrs. Twigg. I shook my head. "Yes, you do," she insisted, her eyes fixed on that non-existent screen, "because they're showing it to me—a small picture, about the size of a passport photograph."

"I don't have one," I replied, "but I wish I did."

"Oh, well, if you don't have one now, you will," she said, confidently, "so make a note of it," pointing to the notebook in which I was writing everything down. "We're not always sure if what we're seeing is the present or the future."

Three months later, I heard from the private investigator in Los Angeles. His report showed that my birth father died a year before my search began; that he had been an alcoholic, and enclosed was a copy of his identification card, which bore a small picture of him—the size of a passport photograph.

With this incident strong in my mind, I reached Jean's office to learn the results of my chlorinated pesticide test.

"The analysis," she began, consulting the report, "shows the presence of DDT and Dieldren, as well as a high level of Heptachlor Epoxide—a very toxic pesticide. Also high are your levels of Beta-BHC."

"What on earth is that?"

"It's a compound of Benzene hexachloride that affects a wide range of enzymes. You also have Hexachlorabenzine, which is found in pesticides, fungicides, and herbicides."

"Oh, no!" I exclaimed, hiding my face in shame. "That wretched spray gun!"

"Highest of all, though," said Jean, "are levels for the herbicides DDE and DDD, which are derivatives of DDT."

"But how can that be? DDT was banned in the U.S. years ago."

"It's banned in the U.K., too," she said, "but these derivatives are being returned to us on the heavily sprayed produce from third world countries, to which they are still being sold.[7]

"Then I must have consumed tons of these toxins, because I've been a vegetarian since 1973."

---

[7] Paul H. Mueller, the Swiss chemist who developed DDT, received a Nobel Prize. Rachel Carson, who warned of its dangers, did not.

"Your pesticide levels aren't as high as those of some other patients," Jean said, reassuringly. "One man's levels are literally off the chart, but you seem to be more sensitive to smaller amounts."

"But how . . . where could I have acquired all these other chemicals?" I asked, bewildered. "The only one I know I was exposed to for years is chlorine."

"You could have absorbed them in a number of ways," she explained. "It needn't always be a strong exposure. The benzenes, for example, are found in dry cleaning fluid, and formaldehyde is found in anything from chipboard (U.S. particle board), to leather goods, to wall insulation."

"But if they're so pervasive they must be impossible to escape," I said.

"I'm afraid so. Commercial products usually contain a combination of several chemicals suspended in a petroleum distillate, as well as a dispensing agent. Exposure to only one is the exception rather than the rule."

So then, the cause of my illness finally was known: I had pesticide poisoning. My symptoms were not psychosomatic; they were *somatopsychic,* as I knew them to be all along. The only question now was—how to get these toxins out of my system?

And could this even be done?

CHAPTER ELEVEN

*The Middle Ages may have been a time of salutary
delay. If it had exploited the earth's surface as we
are doing, we would perhaps not be around at all.*
                                    —Jakob Burckhardt

A conference on allergy was held in London that spring
of 1984. The speakers were Dr. Theron Randolph, Dr. John
Lassiter (the biochemist who developed the chlorinated
pesticide test), and Dr. William Rae, a clinical ecologist from
Dallas, whose Environmentally Controlled Unit (ECU) was
modeled on the one Randolph created for his patients in
Chicago. Of the three addresses, I found Dr. Lassiter's the
most compelling—a cautionary tale about how the
proliferation of chemicals has spread to the farthest reaches
of the Arctic Sea.

"We have put down our probes in the deepest, most
remote parts of the ocean," he said, "and have found that
even there, no part of the sea is any longer free of pollution."

At a dinner given by Jean after the conference, I had the
honor of sitting next to Dr. Randolph, who proved to be the
soul of avuncular warmth. Dr. Rae, a spare, genial man in his
forties, had a back problem, which required him to carry a
special cushion to sit on when he traveled.

Invited by Dr. Lassiter to lunch the next day, I confided
to him my concern that the antigens, which were so helpful
at first, no longer seemed to work. My hay fever had
returned—a disappointment after the sneeze-free season of

the year before—and while the calluses on my feet had healed, some of my former symptoms were creeping back.

"Do you think a two-week stay at Randolph's ECU in Chicago would help?" I asked. "At least it might give my body a rest from the problems I can't seem to escape here in London."

"If I were you," he advised, "I would go to Dr. Rae. He's younger and has newer ideas. If you decide to go to Dallas, tell Rae I sent you—you'll get in quicker."

Adding to my misery that spring were the renovations being carried out in the buildings on either side of number Seven. Lorries dumped their materials on the pavement below, airborne toxins found their way into the flat through the closed windows and particulates drifted down the chimney into my sitting room, depositing a delicate film over the furniture.

As my health continued its downward slide, the square outside my window was burgeoning with life. How I envied nature's ability to renew herself each spring. If the crocus and daffodil could regenerate, why couldn't my hair follicles do the same? According to the Buddhists, everything that lives has once been our mother; therefore, all nature should be respected. But I *did* respect nature, I *loved* her. I cherished every leaf, tree, plant, shrub, and blade of grass in London's gracious parks and squares. So what kind of mother mucks up your sinuses each spring with her pollen?

In July, my heart began to act up again—so violently one evening that, convinced I was having a heart attack, I called Jean.

"Go to the clinic immediately," she ordered. "I'll tell them you're coming and to give you a sleeping pill."

By the time I arrived, however, the arrhythmic heartbeats were settling down, so I declined the sedative. If my heart was going to pack up for good, I wanted to be conscious, not comatose, at the end. Death was too important an adventure to sleep through.

On the 28th, Clive rang for a report on his latest control and we had our first row.

"I don't feel altogether comfortable with it, Clive. It seems to make my heart act funny and my chest feel tight. Do you think the gemstones could be interacting with other crystals somewhere in the building?"

"Nonsense!" he said. "I've had three new controls here in my study for days, each one different, and they haven't bothered me a bit, so whatever you think you're feeling must be in your mind."

To hear from Clive's lips the same dismissive words I'd been hearing from doctors made me grind my teeth. How like him to assume that if *he* couldn't feel an energy that was bothering *me,* it didn't exist—until, of course, it began to bother *him.*

"But you're not as sensitive to crystals as I am," I protested. "You know that."

"As for your heart," he said, ignoring my comment, "I won't even consider that possibility unless you agree to see my wife's heart specialist in Windsor."

"But I don't *have* a heart problem, Clive," I reminded him. "My EKG weeks ago was normal. This tachycardia must be an allergic reaction to something—either some chemical in the flat or one of the crystals."

At this, a small explosion erupted at the other end. Open-minded though he was about most things, Clive was allergic to the mere mention of allergy.

"Anyway," I continued, "I'm not going to waste money on another specialist who will just prescribe Inderal and charge me a whacking great fee."

"Then you will have to leave your flat!" he said, his high-pitched voice rising higher as the line from Maidenhead hotted up. "Why don't you move to the country?"

"And be poisoned by a farmer spraying his crops? No, thank you. I've moved once and that didn't help. It's no use, Clive. Unless I can get these chemicals out of my system, this problem will follow me wherever I go."

"Then I can't help you if you won't take my advice," he said, writing me off in a voice that sounded even stiffer than his neck. "I only deal with the environment."

And on that note he rang off, leaving me with a knot in my stomach that stayed there for the rest of the day. Later that morning, I became aware of a strong chemical odor in the bathroom. It returned briefly that afternoon while I was in the kitchen.

The next morning, I was woken by the sound of clanging pipes at the far end of the flat. I threw on a robe and went to investigate. A scaffold was being erected against the kitchen wall. I raised the window and asked a workman what it was for.

"We're painting the exterior trim," he explained.

Two days later, vapors from an asphalt-making machine in the street made their way into the flat. It was the hottest day of the year and I couldn't open a window because of the fumes. Even the *air* was unfit for human consumption!

The following morning, I was jolted out of bed by the sound of a pneumatic drill. I stumbled to the window and saw some men tearing up the street in the same place they'd torn it up six months before. Every demolition crew in SW7[8] seemed to have descended on Onslow Gardens. Short of ripping up the square, I reckoned, there's not much more they can do.

There was.

That afternoon, they began resurfacing the street—the part they had just ripped up. Fumes from a simmering cauldron snaked their way into my flat, bypassing the air purifier I bought to absorb them. Between the clanging pipes, the asphalt machine, and the hammering that had started up on the other side of the wall, I might have been living in the maw of some cosmic dental patient whose cavities were all being drilled into at once.

Which of all the toxins would be the one to do me in, I wondered: the fumes from the street? The gas-fired paint

---

[8] The Kensington area where I lived.

stripper being used on a neighbor's door? Or her sickening perfume, which hung in the stairwell each time she went out or came in?

Convinced that chemicals were stalking me at every turn, I rang Jean to request an emergency appointment. Sitting in the safety of her office, I tried to describe the building site I inhabited and the feeling that my nervous system was being transferred to the outside of my skin. At one point, I became so overwhelmed by the hopelessness of it all I broke down in tears.

"We must test you for building materials," said Jean, compassionately. "Why don't you come to Greece with us in September? Dr. Rae and I are starting a conference center there and I'll be taking a group of ten patients. It would do you good to get away and the air there would be so much cleaner."

Not in Athens, it wouldn't be, I wanted to say. Why was escape the only answer anyone had to offer? At best, it could give only temporary relief. Persuaded that chemicals would pursue me even to the Aegean, I declined Jean's offer and returned home, more discouraged than ever.

When I arrived, I saw a huge truck marked "Hydrochloric Acid" double-parked in front of the building two doors away. I opened the front door and encountered a new odor in the entrance hall. Seeing the caretaker there, I asked him if he knew what it was.

"It's probably coming from the penthouse," he replied. "They had their carpets cleaned yesterday, and I guess the smell has come down through the stairs."

Then that could account for the sleepless night I spent, I thought, and for that humiliating breakdown in Jean's office, of which I was now ashamed—I, for whom tears were normally so hard to shed.

The following day, I tested for building materials: dry rot, diesel fuel, soft woods, cement and tobacco—strong reactions to all. Arriving home, I saw workmen shoveling what looked like sand into the basement flat next door. How many chemicals had I inhaled from that renovation alone? I

71

wondered—especially from the formaldehyde foam insulation in the walls they were breaking through, which found their way through the chimney into my flat.

The next day, I spotted the caretaker outside talking with Ron, the works manager for the renovation. After greeting them, I said, "Ron, when did the demolition work on your site begin?"

"We started on January 16th," he said.

That meant six months of pollution from his building, with three months from the one on the other side.

Two days later, I thought I detected a familiar odor in the entrance hall. Finding Ron there with a workman, I said, "Do you know what the odor is here in the hall?"

"What odor?" asked Ron.

"You mean you can't smell it? It's similar to the one that comes through that hole in the wall outside my flat."

"Oh, that," he said. "It must be the Cuperdal we've been putting on the timber for the door frames next door."

"We don't smell it, you see," explained the workman, "because we work with it all day long."

But that's why it's so dangerous! I wanted to say. Instead, I said, "You know, you really should wear protective masks when working with such strong chemicals."

"Come to think of it," said Ron, "I've had a headache for several weeks. I wonder if that could be the reason."

"Well, the stuff must be safe," said the workman. "If it wasn't, we'd have been told to wear masks, or been given protective gloves, or something, wouldn't we?"

Two months later, Ron told me he'd been diagnosed with cancer.

CHAPTER TWELVE

"No pain, no gain" is nonsense; pain is not a
badge of honor, it is a sign of tissue injury.
—Berton Rouché

Thanks to the antigens for building materials, my symptoms eased considerably over the summer. By September, however, my legs were aching, my scalp felt funny, and my heart was acting skittish again. More worrying were the two broken toes on my right foot; the bones rubbed painfully against the leather each time I wore proper shoes. There was also a bunion to contend with.

Resigned to the fact that something had to be done, I consulted my new GP, who sent me to a foot surgeon whom I shall call Mr. Baer. I dreaded the thought of another operation—not because I feared surgery, but because the anesthetic would add still more chemicals to my overloaded system. Still, if I wanted to remain ambulatory, I had no choice.

Mr. Baer was a blunt, muscular version of the more austere Dr. Thorne, with pepper-and-salt hair, eyes that looked as though they had never smiled and an impatient manner that forestalled all but the most urgent question. He examined my toes and described the procedure he would perform.

"Now, I shall insert a steel pin in your big toe to keep it straight while it heals," he began, "and in the other toes . . . ."

"Oh, I'm afraid I can't have the pin, Mr. Baer," I broke in. "You see, I'm chemically sensitive and my body will reject a foreign substance."

"Nonsense," he said. "You cannot possibly be allergic to the pin. It's stainless steel, which is inert. It's all in your mind."

I drew a deep breath. "Why would my mind want to make my body suffer?" I asked. He gave me a sour look. I described my experience with the silicone breast implant, but from the expression on his face I might have been explaining metaphysics to a butcher.

"If you refuse to have the pin," Baer warned me, "I cannot be responsible for the outcome. Furthermore," he added, in a faintly threatening manner, "if you don't have the pin, you'll have to wear a cast for at least four weeks to keep your toes immobilized."

"Fine," I said. "I'll be happy to."

This knocked him off his perch for a moment, but he rallied and his manner hardened. Had I been more perceptive, I might have sensed the enmity our exchange had aroused. But I assumed he was just one more doctor for whom environmental illness is a female delusion.

On coming to in the recovery room after the operation I could not believe the pain throbbing in my toes. How could such tiny bones cause such monumental agony? Painkillers gave partial relief, but when I begged the nurse for more she refused. "You've been given the maximum dose allowed," she said, firmly. So I spent the night rocking and moaning in my hospital bed, convinced the pain would never end. Compared to this "minor" intervention, the mastectomy ten years earlier was a lark.

The next day I went home with a knee-high cast and a pair of crutches, to which I easily adapted. The mechanics of living would have been far more difficult, however, had it not been for the kindness of my upstairs neighbor—a fellow American who, seeing me with my sticks in the hall, offered to do my grocery shopping for me, when she did her own.

I was managing quite well when, nine days later, my foot felt as though it was swelling inside the cast. Suspecting the nylon sutures, I made an appointment to see Mr. Baer and ask him to take them out.

"Absolutely not," he said. "The sutures must remain, or your toes won't heal properly."

"I understand that, Mr. Baer, but I know I'm reacting to the nylon and it's causing my foot to swell."

"I've told you," he said, in that how-dare-you-know-more-about-your-body-than-I-do voice, "nylon is inert. You cannot possibly be affected by the sutures."

I did not like Mr. Baer.

"Is there no way I can persuade you to take them out?" I pleaded.

"None," he said.

This threw me into confusion. I knew the nylon was the cause, but was too ashamed of my freakish body—and too intimidated by Baer's authority—to stand up to him. Within hours of returning home, my foot was screaming, "Get these things out of my toes!"

Two days later the swelling had spread to my ankle and by the next morning, my swollen calf was pressing against the cast. Emboldened by fear, I went to see Mr. Baer again on the 28th, determined this time to *make* him remove the stitches.

"After all," I pointed out, "the cast will be coming off anyway in a week."

"Under no circumstance will I remove the cast *or* the sutures," he said, as if I had asked him to remove his clothes.

"But I can feel my leg is swelling, Mr. Baer. Please, *please,* take them out," I begged. "I can't stand the pressure, truly I can't!"

"I'm warning you," he said. "If I remove the cast before time, you will have to remain on crutches for another two weeks."

"I don't care," I cried. "Just take the them out now!"

Baer studied me for a moment with something akin to contempt. Then he picked up the phone and rang the Brompton Hospital to book a room for the following day.

Arriving at the Brompton, I was shown to a cubicle off an open ward and told to wait there for the surgeon. He arrived with a young assistant in tow, gave me a perfunctory greeting and instructed me to lie down on the table. While the assistant arranged some instruments on a tray, I studied the pattern in the curtain he had drawn to screen our cubicle from the communal room beyond.

Baer selected a tool from the tray and began to cut through the plaster cast. I waited expectantly, wondering what he would say when he saw the proof of my swollen calf. I heard the final crack of the plaster and felt the cast fall away from my leg, but from Baer there came not a word. He handed the broken pieces to his acolyte and the next thing I knew, he was ripping the stitches from my toes with such venom, I thought my foot was being raped.

Screaming with pain, I begged him to stop, but Baer went on pulling and tearing, like a deaf butcher trussing a piece of meat on a block. I so hated him in that moment I wished him violently dead. How gladly I would have driven a stake through his heart, if he'd had one!

Mortified that my screams could be heard throughout the ward, I tried to slide off the table, but the assistant held me down. By the time Baer removed the last stitch, I was so shaken I could hardly speak.

"Why didn't you stop when I begged you to?" I said, livid with fury.

He gave me a thin, token smile, like a modern Mengele, but said nothing.

"*Well?*" I demanded.

"Well," Baer replied, with the air of one who has put an opponent out of action, "you said you didn't want an anesthetic."

"You *know* I didn't mean a *local* one!" I shot back. "You might at least have asked or stopped when I begged you to."

But Baer affected not to hear. Collecting his things, he consigned the cast-making job to his assistant, said good-bye and left, leaving me lying on the table, limp with shock and trembling with rage.

The next morning the swelling was gone, and so was my fury of the day before. I was too glad to be rid of the nylon—and too grateful for the relief—to waste my energy cursing Baer and his butchery. Untroubled by the added weeks of restricted mobility, I was managing quite well when, five days later, my foot once more started to swell. How could this be? The sutures were gone and it couldn't be the plaster cast. Unwilling to confront the surgeon again, I went to the emergency room at the Brompton Hospital, prepared to tough it out with Baer on the phone, if necessary.

"I'm sorry," said the young doctor on duty, "but I'm not allowed to remove the cast without the consent of your surgeon. If you wish, I can ring him to ask his permission."

He returned to report that Baer was in the operating theater that morning and would not be in his office until some time after lunch. "I've left a message for him to ring me here, but it could be several hours before he returns the call. Do you want to wait?"

"All day, if necessary," I replied.

For three hours, I sat in the large waiting room watching the walking wounded come and go, while trying to read the Tibetan Book of the Dead. At length, I saw the young doctor heading toward me and knew that a verdict was at hand.

"Mr. Baer has given his consent for the cast to be removed," he announced.

Astonished, and weak with relief, I could only assume that Baer was either heartily sick of me by now or he no longer gave a damn—or both. The young doctor proceeded to remove the cast. With careful fingers he gently unwound the bloody gauze from around my toes. As he lifted the last bit he paused, peered at my foot and said, "Hello, there's a suture here in one toe. Would you like me to take it out?"

"Yes, please," I said, stifling the impulse to cheer.

So I *did* have a guardian angel after all—moreover, one with perfect timing! Would Baer have told me the suture was there if *he'd* been the one to remove the cast? Had he left it on purpose to prove a point, or did he overlook it during the rape? I neither knew nor cared. I knew only that my funny old body had proved again that its warnings could be trusted. *Clever you!* I thought, admiringly, while a smaller cast was fitted to my foot. *You knew it was there, didn't you. I didn't.*

By evening the swelling was gone and I stalked about happily on my sticks for another fortnight. So what if my toes didn't heal as perfectly as they would have done with the pins? At least my body had proved that inert matter can be very *"ert"* indeed.

CHAPTER THIRTEEN

*I hold one share in the corporate earth
and am uneasy about the management.*
—E.B. White

By December 1984, I was still stuck on that frustrating plateau with symptoms that had returned and antigens that no longer worked. With Jean's approval, I flew to Dallas on the 18th, hoping to find in Dr. Rae's ECU some of the answers that eluded me in London.

Dr. Rae greeted me cordially, read the note I presented from Jean, and ordered blood to be drawn for a round of tests. After waiting several hours for another new patient to arrive and be checked in, I was driven with her to the ECU, which occupied one floor of a hospital twenty minutes away.

Before we could enter the unit we had to pass through an antechamber, where we relinquished our personal effects and exchanged our clothes for the white cotton scrub suits that were to be our uniform for the next two weeks. The door to the unit was as thick as a bank vault's and bore the familiar sign forbidding entry to anyone wearing perfume, make-up, hair spray, or shaving lotion.

Once admitted, we found ourselves in a spotless world of tiled floors, stainless steel walls, and furnishings that were sparse, but serviceable—and safe. Vents in the ceiling delivered a steady flow of filtered air, the constant hum adding to the feeling of being on a spaceship as it floats through the cosmos.

The only writing materials allowed were a stenographer's pad and a lead pencil. Our only books were those old enough to have lost the smell of print, while not yet old enough to have acquired the scent of mold. Taped to the wall above the scale on which we weighed ourselves each morning was a large square of aluminum foil, into which a patient had laboriously punched out the words:

We are all faced with brilliant opportunities,
brilliantly disguised as insurmountable problems.

Each evening, Dr. Rae arrived to make his rounds, accompanied by Dr. Evans, the young physician who was on duty during the day. In the large testing room a lone nurse was doing her best to cope with twenty-six patients. There should have been three nurses on duty, but because of the Christmas holiday, the unit was short-staffed.

Reactions to the antigens were familiar. Some patients grew sleepy when challenged, some grew hyperactive, while others, injected with the same substance, became irascible or depressed. One woman grew tearful when testing for Orrisroot—a component of perfume, hair spray, and shaving cream, while two patients wore charcoal masks even in the unit.

"We're affected by the electronic equipment at the nurses' station," they explained.

One could sympathize with doctors who might feel the problem had more to do with their minds than their molecules, but my heart went out to them—and to all the other sufferers I met, most of whom had immune systems far more damaged than mine.

And yet, when I saw that, even after weeks of testing, some patients still could not tolerate more than a few foods, I began to question the long-term validity of the antigen approach. Surely, the body needs a variety of nutrients if it is to heal, let alone survive.

While discussing my symptoms with Dr. Evans the first day, I described for him the feeling of an acid creeping under my scalp.

"I know," he nodded. "It's like a headache."

"It is not in the least like a headache," I said, bristling at the glib reply. Good grief, I thought; if a clinical ecology doctor can't be curious, what am I doing here?

"It's just that—it's such a peculiar symptom," he said, lamely, as though that absolved him of the need even to try find the cause.

"Of course, it's peculiar," I said. "We're all peculiar here."

"Well," he hedged, backing away from the problem and toward the door, "let's see how you get on with the double-blind chemical tests—and the fast."

The chemical booth formed part of a small area that included a changing room, a shower and a heart-monitoring machine. Although some of the tests would involve a placebo, the shower and shampoo were obligatory after each one, since a trace of the chemical could remain on the skin. I exchanged my scrub suit for a cotton kimono and entered the booth. A young technician, Debbie, took my blood pressure, gave me a pulmonary test and attached electrodes to my chest and legs.

"You're to take your pulse three times during the ten-minute test," said Debbie, after showing me how. "Then give me the reading and report any symptoms you may have."

She placed a canister on the floor, instructing me to unscrew the cap of the bottle inside after she left. "The unlabeled bottle contains either a placebo or a chemical, which you will breathe for a certain period of time," she explained.

She closed the hermetically sealed door and took up her post by the table with the monitoring equipment. A window in the door allowed her to observe my reactions, while we communicated through an intercom.

There were six tests in all. At the end of each one, I was to return to my room and record my pulse rate at fifteen-minute intervals for an hour, together with any symptoms that might appear. The first bottle caused no reaction, so I assumed it was a placebo. The second bottle released an odor that resembled nail varnish or paint. My nose clogged up and I felt dizzy and sneezed. The third one was neutral, but with the fourth, while I couldn't identify the odor, I grew light-headed and garrulous with Debbie.

In my room, my hands developed a slight tremor, which spread to my thighs and culminated in a mild panic attack. By the time Debbie came by two hours later, the symptoms had gone.

"I could tell you were hyper on that last test," she said, "because you became very loquacious, and you're not normally the chatty type. You seem to be calmer within yourself than most of the people we see here."

"What was the chemical?" I asked, eagerly.

"Sorry," she said, "I'm not allowed to say."

Later, I learned it was formaldehyde.

Environmentally ill patients know from experience that long-term, low-grade toxicity can result in a hyper-acute sense of taste, hearing or smell. The smallest whiff of fragrance in the ECU's purified air was like an assault on my hyperactive hippocampus. Twice, I suspected a nurse of using perfume, which was forbidden in the unit. In each case, the nurse in question had washed her hair the night before, and it was the trace of phthalates in the shampoo rinse that triggered a reaction in my twitchy olfactory nerves. Hard though it was to live with such exaggerated acuity, it did at least warn us of the things we needed to avoid.

Dr. Rae stressed this one evening, when he advised us not to go into public places for several weeks after we leave the unit.

"You will be extremely vulnerable for a while," he warned. "Inhalants such as phenol, formaldehyde, and tobacco smoke are pervasive in enclosed areas such as malls, drug stores and department stores. The rule is: If you can smell it, avoid it."

I thought of the obstacle course I had to run each time I went to Harrods to avoid being sprayed with scent by a roaming predator from the perfume counter.

On December 20th, the four-day fast began. I weighed 121 pounds and couldn't wait to begin. What I loathed most about my affliction was that it forced me to make food the focus of my life. I didn't want to think about food—*or* my body—fourteen hours a day. The prospect of a four day fast, therefore, seemed like very heaven.

The first day left me feeling weak and muddled. On the second, I rallied, but on the third, I woke with a headache. Dr. Evans came by to tell me the chemical tests showed that my allergies were primarily chemical, which I already knew. By the fourth fasting day I had lost eight pounds, my symptoms were gone and I had so much energy I felt I could levitate.

Christmas Day dawned bleak and beautiful, the whitened world outside my window as surreal as the one in which I was temporarily cocooned. The 25th also marked the end of the fast and the beginning of single-food meals. Patients were allowed to choose the one food they would eat each day, so I chose baked apple. I had consumed no more than half when my fingers turned red, my scalp woke up, and my heart began to do a funny jig.

It was the same each day no matter which food I chose. I recalled Randolph telling me about patients whose symptoms vanished after a five-day fast, only to return when a drop of an allergen was placed under their tongue. How, then, could fasting either help or cure?

It didn't help that the food was badly cooked and kept in a warming compartment until mealtime. When patients complained about the half-cooked rice swimming in a bowl of glutinous liquid (to cite but one example), we were told it was because a temporary staff was on duty over Christmas.

On the 26th, Dr. Rae came by on his regular round. I described for him the return of my symptoms the day I began the single-food meals.

"I'm sure it's just an allergy that will clear up if you stay on the rotation diet," he said.

On hearing the words, "rotation diet," I groaned. I had tried the Rotary Diversified Diet the year before, but gave it up after six months—not because it was wrong, but because of the time it took to prepare all the foods that had to be stored in the freezer and eaten in a certain order. The principle of the diet is to consume the widest possible variety of foods in order to control existing allergies and prevent the formation of new ones.

Because the transit time through the human digestive system requires up to three days, no single food can be repeated within four days—a tricky task if one is a vegetarian. It became even trickier when I found that certain vegetables belong to the same family—not just logical ones, such as cauliflower, broccoli and sprouts, but peculiar ones, such as potato, eggplant and tomato. This meant that I had to avoid *every* family member for four days.

Sticking a chart of these ancestral trees on my kitchen wall, I was dismayed to discover how many of my favorite vegetables belong to the same clan. The diet was a gastronomic seat belt—safe, but restricting—and the thought of doing all that cooking, wrapping, dating, and storing again, sent my spirits tumbling into a black hole. When, oh when, would I ever have time to *write?*

"Meanwhile," said Dr. Rae, "I think you should leave London and go live somewhere by the sea."

Had I come all this way, I wondered, and spent all this money, only to receive from Rae the same advice Jean and Clive had been giving me for free? Although the tests confirmed *what* I was reacting to, there was still no program for getting the chemicals out of my system.

The day I left the ECU's pure environment, I found I was even more sensitive than the day I went in. It took so short a time to forget what the world was like—the noise, the pollution, the perfume—that the shock of reentry was seismic. The moment I stepped into the hospital corridor, its odors knocked me sideways. I paid my bill and rushed outside, gasping for air—or rather, air less contaminated than the chemical soup inside. Was I doomed to spend the rest of my life in this pan-reactive state?

I thought of the so-called lesser animals, whose very survival depends on their delicate sense of smell. Given the toxic fog in which we have surrounded ourselves, we are destroying not only our own early warning system, but theirs as well. When we can no longer see, hear, sense, or smell the enemy, it is already within the gates.

CHAPTER FOURTEEN

One must be taught to suspect, for if one
Does not suspect, one does not test, and
If one does not test, one does not know.
—*Dr. Herbert Rinkell*

Before leaving the ECU, I asked Dr. Rae about some
dental work I needed to have done. It concerned an
automobile accident I had thirty years before. Of the accident
I had only the haziest recollection: a light drizzle on the
winding road, the sudden swerve to avoid a car pulling out
from the curb and a large tree racing toward me from the
opposite side of the street.

When I regained consciousness I was in the hospital with
a broken jaw and a jagged gash under my lower lip, where
some perfect teeth made their exit. The car was a write-off
and my escape with only a fractured mandible deemed a
miracle by the Catholic nurse in attendance: "You must have
had an angel on your shoulder!"

A remarkable dentist in Beverly Hills devised a precision
attachment bridge (actually a partial) of such ingenuity, that
for thirty-five years it elicited awe from every dentist who
peered into my mouth, from New York City to Rome and
from Paris to London. Given the normal changes that occur
in the mouth over time, the bridge needed to be replaced.
Newly aware of the perils lurking in dentistry for the
chemically sensitive, and uncertain of finding a "safe"
dentist in London, I asked Dr. Rae if he knew someone in

Dallas skilled enough to duplicate the partial that had served me well for so long.

"I know an excellent dentist," he said, "but you must warn him not to use epinephrine in the anesthetic." Surely he would know this if he has treated E.I. patients, I thought. "Epinephrine provides the staying power," Rae explained, "so without it, you'll need more frequent injections. If you decide to have the work done here, a patient of mine has a 'safe house' where you can stay as a paying guest. Let me know and I'll find out if Willie Mae has an available room."

Willie Mae Phipps was a widow in her late sixties: grey hair escaping from a hair net, beige cardigan flung over a flowered housedress, white ankle socks, brown carpet slippers and the kind of Texas drawl that did funny things to her vowels. An ardent Baptist, she kept her kitchen radio glued to one of the many religious stations in Dallas, which provided a gospel-thumping backdrop to mealtime conversations. Pictures of angels in various postures of prayer adorned her walls, with pride of place held by a huge plate inscribed with *The Lord's Prayer* that hung over her kitchen table.

Since I possessed only the sketchiest knowledge of Baptist belief, I asked Willie Mae about its tenets one day while she was peeling potatoes in the kitchen.

"You gotta be saved," she said, flatly, chucking potato skins into the compost basket. "If you don't accept Jesus Christ as your Lord, you cain't be saved. When you die, you'll be judged and be sent straight down to Hell."

Hell or no, Willie Mae extended her hospitality to saved and sinner alike, for whom the toxic perils in an average hotel would have been akin to purgatory. When I arrived on the 4th of January, I found another patient already installed. Louise was tall, thin, pale, and on the cusp of forty. She had been an administrative official at a school when someone emptied cleaning fluid down the drain of a supply room across the hall from her office. Without knowing why, she became ill and disoriented, her body went into spasms and she couldn't eat.

"No one knew what was wrong with me," she said. "I fell into a coma and went blind for a while. Months later, when I recovered enough to return to work, I was exposed to *another* chemical accident. This time, my immune system was virtually destroyed. If I held a telephone receiver against my ear, I felt sharp pains shooting through my head. The doctors thought I was loopy, of course, but when I had the amalgam fillings removed from my teeth, that particular phenomenon disappeared."[9]

After twenty days of antigen testing, Louise could eat only nine foods without suffering an allergic reaction, although she should have had a minimum of sixteen. Odors that I could tolerate wiped her out, especially those that abound in public places. If she had to enter a store or fly in a plane, she wore a grotesque charcoal mask that made her look like a deep-sea diver or an alien from outer space. Even my "unscented" face powder bothered her, so I abstained from using it while there.

"The reason I sleep here in the kitchen on a folding bed is because I couldn't tolerate the mold in that upstairs bedroom," Louise explained, referring to the room I had just inherited. "It's truly awful."

Mold wasn't the half of it. The rectangular room had a bed at one end, while stacked at the opposite end were pieces of furniture that looked as though they hadn't been moved for years. Large sheet-covered boxes lined the wall on my left, while directly opposite, hanging from a portable clothes rack, were vintage garments lightly mantled with dust..

Safe house, indeed. Had Rae ever vetted it or had he taken Willie Mae's word that her home was free of allergens? It may have been safe for her, but toxins one person can tolerate may devastate another. At least I could

---

[9] The first argument within the dental profession about the dangers of mercury amalgam fillings occurred as early as 1840, and has been resisted by the establishment ever since.

do something about those tumbleweeds of dust under the bed.

My first night in the room, the thermometer fell to 20 degrees Fahrenheit and the electric heater didn't work.

"You'll have to pay extra for heat," said Willie Mae the next morning, when I complained of the cold. It took three days for the heater to be repaired. Whether it was the mold, the dust, or the perishing cold, throughout my four weeks' stay at Willie Mae's I had chronic rhinitis.

On the 6th of January, I met with Dr. Rae to discuss the chemical analyses of the two blood samples that were taken the day I arrived.

"One shows moderate levels of pentaphenol and chlorophenol in the serum," he said, consulting the report, "as well as styrene and benzene."

"What does pentaphenol do?" I asked. "It doesn't sound body-friendly."

"It's used in treating wood and leathers, things such as shoes and handbags."

"And where could I have acquired the styrene?"

"That would have come from breathing fumes given off by packing materials, or from drinking out of styrene cups, hot liquids especially."

"Which I never do."

"Of greater concern, though," said Rae, "is the test for volatiles, which shows a high amount of methylene chloride."

"My, that sounds ominous. Where would that have come from?"

"From inhaling the propellant in aerosol cans, for instance, such as those used for pesticides." Oh, no! I thought, those bug-killing sprees again! "Of course," Rae added, "you would have been more susceptible to methylene chloride if you had other chemicals in your body, which you do. What makes it more worrisome is that you wear contact lenses."

"Why contact lenses?" I asked, surprised.

"Because they absorb strong vapors and hold them against your eyes, which can cause irritation or damage. The worst problem with methylene chloride, however, is the way it combines with hemoglobin in the blood to create carbon monoxide. This prevents the blood from carrying oxygen to the tissues." More chemicals to worry about then, and still no way to get them out of my system.

A week had gone by before I realized that the supplements I should have been taking, as well as the results of my other tests, hadn't arrived. When I rang Rae's office to inquire, I learned they had been sent to London. No one had thought to inform them I would be staying on for a month. By the time I got home, I had missed four weeks of supplements that might, or might not, have forestalled the ongoing collapse of my immune system.

On the 7th of January I met the dentist Dr. Rae recommended, whom I shall call Dr. Benson. A soft-spoken, likeable man, he examined my partial and said he could replicate it if I would leave it with him and make do with the spare. After taking X-rays of my mouth, he found some decay under two teeth and mercury amalgam under two fillings.

"I'm afraid that to remove the amalgam and deal with the decay, I will have to redo the precision inlays on both sides." he said. He was also concerned about a root canal on the lower left side that had bothered me for years. "I'm concerned because formaldehyde is usually poured into the root to numb the nerve, and then it continues to leech into the gums. It really should be removed."

This was a bad surprise; I hadn't expected such extensive work to be required. Dr. Benson gave me an appointment for the 10th and I returned to Willie Mae's in time to see a large oxygen tank being delivered to the house.

"It's for Betty," said Willie Mae, "the patient who's arriving tonight from New Jersey. She's extremely sensitive and always stays with me when she comes here for treatment with Dr. Rae."

I heard Betty's arrival downstairs at half past ten that night, but we didn't meet until lunch the next day. A lively, attractive brunette in her forties, she, too, had suffered a series of chemical insults that virtually destroyed her immune system.

"After working in an aircraft assembly plant for several years," she said, "I was affected by the chemicals, so I found a job in the safer environment of an office. Unfortunately, new carpeting had been installed. The chemicals that outgassed from the carpet and underlay further weakened my immune system." An accident at work, similar to the one Louise had suffered, dealt her body the final blow. "It's left me hypersensitive to certain foods," Betty explained, "which is why I need to have oxygen nearby in case of an emergency."

Minutes later, Betty suddenly dropped her fork, pointed to the mashed potatoes Willie Mae made for us and gasped, "Is there butter in this?"

"Only a smidgen," said Willie Mae, looking alarmed.

"I've got to have oxygen!" cried Betty, stumbling from the table and running to her room.

"I forgot she cain't tolerate butter," said Willie Mae, looking stricken.

Dismayed, we sat in worried silence, moving the food around on our plates, our thoughts troubled, our appetites gone. Contemplating the loneliness of pain and the way suffering isolates us, one from the other, I thought of something Edith Hamilton wrote in *The Greek Way:*

> Pain is the most individualizing thing on earth . . . To suffer is to be alone. To watch another suffer is to know the barrier that shuts each of us away by himself.

When Betty returned, she showed us her swollen fingers and the palms of her hands, which were now rough and cracked.

"This is what happens when I'm having a reaction," she explained. "If I eat anything with butter in it, my whole body goes haywire. My fingers swell up and I become incoherent and act like a crazy woman. Ten minutes on my oxygen tank with a shot of serotonin, and I'm almost normal again."

How infinitely diverse are the stigmata of allergy, I reflected.

Desperately in need of exercise, and with my next dental appointment three days away, I realized I hadn't brought any walking shoes, since they weren't needed in the ECU. Forgetting Rae's warning about public places, I decided to go to a nearby mall and look for the shoes. Scarcely had I entered the building when my body cried *panic stations!* Reeling from all the odors in the concourse, I bought the first comfortable shoes I could find and fled the mall with them on.

Walking back to Willie Mae's, I was pleased to find my emergency purchase surprisingly comfortable. After a while, however, I felt a mild burning around the instep. As soon as I removed the shoes at home the burning stopped, but when I wore them the next day, the same thing happened.

I was describing this oddity at dinner that evening, when Betty said, "Let me see the shoes."

"Oh, they're all leather," I assured her, anticipating her concern as I went to fetch one.

Holding the shoe in one hand, Betty felt around the interior with the other. Then she peered inside.

"They may be leather on the outside," she said, handing the shoe back to me, "but the interlining feels like acrylic. I'll bet that's what's affecting you—that, and your nylon stockings."

So eager had I been to escape the mall, I hadn't noticed the shiny mesh lining inside the shoe—nor would I have questioned it if I had, for it covered the soft padding that made the shoe so comfortable.

"The reason I spotted it," said Betty, "is because once, when I bought a new cotton dress, I couldn't understand why

I felt uncomfortable every time I wore it. Eventually, suspecting the nylon label in the back, I cut it out, and after that the dress was fine. So I removed the nylon labels from all my clothes."

"That's why people think we're crazy," said Louise, who knew from long experience. "They don't understand that when the immune system breaks down, virtually anything can cause a strong reaction, no matter how crazy it seems."

"The trouble is," said Willie Mae, "most doctors don't know any more about chemical illness than we do ourselves."

"That's right," said Betty. "Sickness has made sleuths of us all. We have to be our own detectives, because doctors don't have time to track down the cause of our problems, and even if they did, few would bother." Turning to me again, she said, "It doesn't look as though that lining stuff can be removed from your shoes. If you wear dark cotton socks, they should protect you."

When I told Dr. Rae about my reaction to the acrylic the next day, he looked surprised.

"It's the first time I've heard of such a peculiar sensitivity," he said.

"Surely not," I replied. "I've seen far stranger sensitivities in the testing room."

But then, Rae could hardly know the reactions of every patient who came to him for help. It was enough that he offered an alternative path for those who had exhausted the conventional route and had nowhere else to turn.

In the end, however, it was not from the doctors in Dallas that I learned the most about environmental illness—it was from Betty and Louise and from all the chemically-damaged patients I met in the ECU.

And it was Betty who, a few days later, gave me the advice that may even have saved my life.

CHAPTER FIFTEEN

Wherever a doctor cannot do good,
He must be kept from doing harm.
　　　　　—Hippocrates

On the 10th of January, Dr. Benson began drilling out the old attachment inlays before tackling the problems of amalgam and decay. "I think you're doing very well with the epinephrine," he said, encouragingly. The next day's session went almost as well as the first, although I needed more frequent injections of anesthetic. Half-way through the third session, however, I began to feel distinctly fragile. By the time he dealt with the last tooth, my nerves were jangled and my head felt as though it was filled with helium.

"Well, that's it," said Benson, rolling away from the chair on his stool. "We're finished. I must say, you've held up better than I expected."

He retreated to the counter behind me to prepare the alginate for the impression tray. Relieved the worst was over I closed my eyes and sank back in the chair, letting the coils of nervous tension unwind. As I drifted into a hypnagogic state, amorphous images rose, merged, and dissolved behind my eyelids. I seemed to be floating in another dimension—light-headed, bodyless and blissfully free.

Suddenly my heart lurched, my blood sugar dropped and I felt the life force drain from my body. *I'm dying!* I thought, surprised. I tried to speak, but no voice came. I tried to move, but the link between body and the brain's command center was cut. Suspended in limbo between life and death, I felt a spasm of real fear.

Dr. Benson reappeared and began to ease the impression tray into my mouth. Even in my parlous state I could see the irony of a mold being made of my teeth while the rest of me was about to expire. By the time he removed the tray, however, I assumed the expiration date was postponed.

Benson retreated again to prepare the cement for the temporary caps. Still too weak to move, I struggled to clear the fog from my brain. At length, my frail strength returning, I managed to say, "Dr. Benson . . . when you were preparing the alginate . . . did you introduce a new substance into the room?"

"No, nothing that wasn't out before. Why?"

"Because I felt as though I . . . ." But the fog closed in again and I grew confused. "Oh, nothing," I said.

My mouth felt dry. I thought of the bottle of mineral water in my bag and tried to rise, but my legs had turned to jelly. By the time Benson finished cementing the temporary caps, my voice had recovered enough to tell him what happened.

"Well, you *have* had a lot of anesthetic today," he said, sympathetically.

Although my strength had returned, I still felt too disoriented to drive home safely, so I decided to wait in the reception room until my head cleared. But shouldn't Benson have suggested this himself? For a dentist familiar with E.I. patients, he was surprisingly clueless about the most elementary precautions. Why, I wondered, did Rae recommend him? Were they golfing chums or did Rae owe him a favor?

At dinner that evening, I was describing my near-death experience in the dental chair, when Betty cut in, her eyes wide with disbelief.

"You mean he didn't have you wear an oxygen mask while he worked on you?"

"No. Why? Should he have?"

"Of course! Sensitive patients should *never* have dental work done without oxygen. I'm surprised he didn't insist on it himself."

"I don't think he knew," I said, feeling stupid—and then alarmed.

"Well, frankly," said Betty, "I think you've had far too much work done on your teeth so soon after leaving the unit. You're too vulnerable to have had all that anesthetic, even without the epinephrine. Why, do you realize," she added, addressing the table, "that all of us on this planet are living with one-third less oxygen today than was originally here? One-third *less* than we should be breathing right now!"

"That wouldn't surprise me," said Louise, "the way we've been cutting down forests and spreading chemicals everywhere." Willie Mae nodded her vigorous agreement.

"Imagine how different we would feel," Betty went on, "if we lived in a world without chemicals and had a third more oxygen to breathe. Why, we would be *amazed* at our sense of well-being!"

Just then, our attention was caught by a news item on the radio, which had been chattering irrelevantly in the background: *"A plant near a major Texas City will soon be manufacturing methyl isocyanate."*

"Isn't that the chemical that devastated Bhopal in India?" I said, the memory of that horror still lingering in my mind.

A silence fell as we listened to the rest of the report, exchanging glances and shaking our heads. Scarcely a week went by without news of a chemical disaster somewhere—a lorry shedding its toxic load on a highway or a tanker spilling its oil into the sea—disasters followed invariably by someone in authority telling us, "There is no immediate danger."

Within hours of a recent chemical spill on the road, drivers in the vicinity were being told, "No one having temporary breathing or eye difficulties will experience any lasting damage." How did they know? On what evidence did they base their assurance? It could be years before the effects of such an exposure surfaced, by which time the cause would

96

be forgotten and it would be too late for victims to sue; too late, as well, for the damage to be undone.[10]

At the end of the report, Betty rose and carried her plate to the sink. Returning to the table, she stood with one hand on her hip, the other resting on the back of her chair.

"Do you know what the most endangered species on this planet really is?" she asked. "It's us. *We're* the human canaries keeling over to warn of the dangers that lie ahead if we keep fouling our nest the way we're doing."

"The trouble is," said Louise, her sad eyes growing sadder, "no one is listening. Besides, who will protect us from the pharmaceutical companies? Not the FDA[11] or the government—not when big Pharma pours millions of dollars into the coffers of both political parties."

"That's right," said Willie Mae. "Most people never suspect their aches and pains, like arthritis, could be caused by chemicals, and are made even worse by all the drugs they're taking. And the doctors cain't tell them, 'cause they don't know themselves."

"And most people don't even care," I said.

"I'll tell you something else," said Betty, her voice crisp with contempt. "We take better care of our *cars* than we do of our bodies!"

Later that evening, while helping Willie Mae with the dishes, I noticed that whenever I touched something metal, like a saucepan, I experienced an odd metallic taste on my tongue. Before going to bed that night, I took a pocket mirror and peered into my mouth. It was as I suspected—the caps on my teeth were metal. No dentist had put metal temporay caps on my teeth before.

---

[10] In July 2007, when a 6.8 earthquake in Japan caused damage far worse than the accident at Three Mile Island, officials initially downplayed the danger. Eventually, it was revealed that 400 barrels of contaminated radioactive materials spilled their contents into the sea, almost 400 gallons of highly toxic waste. Additionally, an undisclosed amount of Cobalt 60 and other dangerous radioactive contaminants escaped into the air, but no warning was given to citizens in the area.

[11] Food and Drug Administration.

Aware that mixed metals create a galvanic reaction in the mouth, I suspected the caps were interacting with a couple of gold inlays. Had I not been dealing with death that last session, I might have noticed what Benson was doing and could have stopped him.

The next morning, I was on the phone to his office as soon as it opened.

"Dr. Benson, the caps you put on my teeth yesterday . . . what are they made of?"

"They're aluminum."

"Aluminum!" I cried. How could anyone with the least knowledge of chemical sensitivity have put aluminum in my mouth? "Well, I think I'm reacting to them."

Hearing the alarm in my voice, Benson said, "I can change them to stainless steel for you, if you want to come in this morning."

I jumped into my rented hatchback and sped to his office—passing on the way a billboard sign that said, "JESUS ALONE IS THE ANSWER!"

Not when you need a good dentist . . . .

"I've never had a patient who was allergic to aluminum before," said Benson, while replacing the offending caps, "but then I don't know much about allergies."

It was too late to wonder why I let him finish the job, when my body had been warning me not to for days. With a sense of foreboding, I drove back to Willie Mae's.

That night, I came down with the flu.

Thanks to Betty's hectoring, for my penultimate post-flu dental appointment I was wearing an oxygen mask. The difference it made was dramatic. Indeed, without oxygen I might well have come to grief, for this time Benson was finding it harder to keep me desensitized.

"I don't know why you're metabolizing more quickly today than you did before," he said.

"I do. It's because I'm full of chemicals."

"Oh, is that it?"

He brought out the new partial to show me and my heart fell. It didn't look like the original. Benson eased it into my mouth and I tested the fit with my fingers.

"It doesn't feel as secure as the old one," I said.

"It just needs a bit of adjusting," he replied, with more confidence than I felt able to share. He removed the partial and worked on it for a few minutes before positioning it again in my mouth.

"It still doesn't feel right," I said, with mounting concern.

"Well, it may take a few days for your teeth to adjust to it," said Benson.

Too late, I knew my misgivings were well-founded. The bridge was a disaster. With a leaden heart, I realized that much of the work would have to be redone in London—if I could find a dentist there willing and able to undo the damage Benson had wrought. Beguiled by the man's evident niceness, I now felt betrayed by his ineptitude. With the best will in the world he had ruined my mouth. Moreover, his ignorance had almost cost me my life.

"Good grief!" exclaimed Betty, when I entered the kitchen. "You look like the stuffing's been knocked out of you, girl. Didn't he give you any oxygen?" I nodded. "Well, then, you need some more. Come with me!" She grabbed my hand and marched me into her room, where she hooked me up to her oxygen cylinder. "Now you stay there until you've fully recovered," she ordered, "do you hear?"

I felt far safer in Betty's hands than I did in those of the dentist. Within minutes my strength was restored, and I returned to the kitchen in time to give Betty a hand with dinner and a grateful hug.

The final session almost did me in, oxygen mask notwithstanding. Each time Benson cemented a tooth, the nerve spasmed with pain. At one point my body warned, *No more anesthetic!* I managed to get through the last half-hour without it, but had it not been for Betty's benevolent bullying, I might not be writing this account today.

"How did he get it so wrong?" I wailed to her that evening. "All he had to do was copy the original, which he had right there in front of his nose the whole time!"

After I returned to London, I found an excellent dentist who managed to correct Benson's worst mistakes. Thanks to his skill he created a serviceable replacement, turning a dental disaster into something I could live with.

Two years later, I received a letter from Louise, telling me the ECU had been closed after a patient died while having some dental work done—presumably after leaving the unit. Whether that was the reason I do not know, but the ECU did close some time after I left.

Sadly, the information came too late to be shared with Betty. A year after my return to England, I learned that she had died.

CHAPTER SIXTEEN

The painful faces asked, can we not cure?
We answer, No, not yet; we seek the laws.
Oh God, reveal thro' all this thing obscure
The unseen, small, but million-murdering cause
—Sir Ronald Ross

I flew home from Dallas on February 24, 1985, holding a charcoal mask over my nose for part of the flight to protect me from the cabin's recycled air.[12] Although I was seated in the nonsmoking section (the total ban was not yet in force), each time I removed the mask the smell of smoke was as strong as if the passenger sitting next to me had lit a cigarette.

On opening the front door at Onslow Gardens I was met by the smell of varnish in the hall; a neighbor was having her parquet floor refinished. *Why, oh why do these poisons pursue me?* I cried out to an indifferent God. To this cry my body responded (since God did not) with a creative new array of symptoms.

I turned on the central heating and thought I could smell the odorless gas. I couldn't, but in bed that night my heart skipped about erratically in my chest. Days later, an EKG showed my heart again to be fine.

---

[12] "Aircraft air can be laced with toxic mixtures of chemicals, such as tricresyl phosphate, that have been linked to serious respiratory problems, memory loss, neurological illnesses, and even brain damage. *The London Daily Telegraph,* February 21, 2008.

With a zeal known only to the terminally allergic, I set about transforming my flat from an ecological threat into a toxin-free oasis—discovering, as I did so, how hard it is, and how expensive, to rely wholly on chemical-free products. Exchanging the few remaining poisonous items under my sink for less contaminating—and less efficient—substitutes, I replaced the bedroom carpet with tile, synthetic fabrics with those of cotton, and gave my new, scarcely worn polyester caftan to Oxfam. About the outside environment, however, I could do nothing.

To the chemicals affecting my respiratory system were added mold and rot from the renovation two doors away. Each time I passed the bags of dry cement stacked in front of the building I experienced a faint nausea—and once, walking in the wake of a woman half a block ahead of me, I picked up a trace of her perfume.

While sifting through the mail that arrived in my absence, I found the supplements that should have been sent to Willie Mae's, along with the confidential results of my tests. These were mailed in envelopes so poorly sealed they could easily have been opened by anyone with an inquisitive eye.

Adding to my discouragement was the thought of all the different foods I was going to have to prepare for the rotation diet. I wanted to *write,* damn it, not cook. All I asked of food was that it be fresh, organic, and uncontaminated.

Meanwhile, in addition to the tachycardia, my brain kept going absent without leave. I caught myself doing mindless things, such as throwing socks into the wastebasket instead of the laundry hamper and searching for objects that, when found, were in front of my nose all the time. Fear of dementia loomed large. As for God, if He happened to be listening, all I asked of *Him* was that He send me an answer soon—in this lifetime, if possible.

In May, I had the gas boiler removed and the central heating changed from gas to electricity, a step recommended by Randolph and Rae. The pipes were capped on the 8th, and by the 12th, it dawned on me that I hadn't had a tachycardia incident since. My hay fever, however, had returned with a vengeance. Either there was more pollen in the air that year, or the antigens no longer worked.

Each time I went to the clinic for an intravenous vitamin C drip, my elusive veins went into hiding at the sight of a needle. Twice, when the nurse couldn't find a vein, she turned me over to Jean, whose expertise invariably found one on the first try. At the end of June, however, when *two* nurses failed after four painful attempts—and this time, not even Jean could find a vein—I knew that clinical ecology had done as much for me as it could.

I had been having doubts about the vaccination approach, at least for me. To neutralize, after all, is not to cure. True, the antigens enabled people to cope with harmful substances they could not avoid, but a body weakened by chemicals needs to be purged of them—not helped to tolerate them, except as a temporary measure. For all its proven benefits, the vaccination method had no program for radical detoxification, and mainstream medicine ignored even the need for one. If my body no longer responded to the homeopathic approach—well, human beings are not a one-cure-fits-all species. But where, then, was the cure for me?

Along with the search for healing, I had been yearning for something to fill the spiritual void that remained when I left the church in 1963. After I moved to England, I began to explore different forms of spirituality in the hope of gaining some insight into life's infinite perplexity. It was the sort of search one undertakes in one's twenties, not one's forties, but I had a lot of catching up to do.

The confirmation of Ena Twigg's clairvoyance convinced me of the soul's survival after death, although that wasn't what I was seeking at all. Still searching, I enrolled in consciousness-raising seminars, such as *Silva Mind Control, Insight,* and *est.* Yet now, when my need for guidance was greater than ever, there seemed to be fewer teachers whose message brought fresh inspiration or whose answers—some of them, at least—I had not found wanting as a result of my own experience. Sometimes, the student returns from his own far journey to find the guru still there, chanting the same mantra or preaching the same sermon—only now, words that once had inspired seem to be frozen in aspic.

"You know," said Clive that summer on one of his visits to London, "I may not be able to solve your problem after all. I've tried everything I can think of, but I'm afraid I've shot my bolt."

I had known for some time that neither Clive nor his crystals could be the answer. Indeed, given their effect on my body, crystals were part of the problem. Yet so addictive had our experiments become, I didn't want them to end.

Much of what sustained me when things looked darkest was the knowledge that Clive—practical, pragmatic, and profoundly leery of mysticism—could validate the cause of my physical torment. He, too, could feel a fractured energy line or confirm the presence of a polluted stream, only he needed a divining rod to find them. If his attempts to neutralize the energies for me had failed, at least he proved their telluric origin. Moreover, his efforts had given me hope when I desperately needed something to cling to. And such is the nature of hope that even false hope can sustain us through trials that, without it, we might not be able to bear.

Two nights after Clive's visit, I found myself again in that familiar hell wherein sanity is destroyed, reason absent, and consciousness splinters into a thousand fragments. Casting about for something to anchor my mind, I reached for the new book on my nightstand. The title was *A Time to Heal,* and its author, Beata Bishop, was a personal friend. The narrative described her healing of malignant melanoma through an unconventional nutritional therapy.

Beata's cancer began as a mole on her shin. When the mole became enlarged, her oncologist diagnosed it as melanoma and it was surgically removed. A painful skin graft followed, but within a year the cancer returned and spread to her groin. Unwilling to submit to a second operation, which offered only a fifty-fifty chance of success, she decided to try the little-known Gerson Therapy, which has a clinic in Mexico.

I had followed Beata's adventure with this unorthodox regime, admiring her courage, while marveling at her ability to adhere to the many strictures it imposed. It did not merely advise reducing salt, sugar, coffee, wheat, meat, alcohol, tobacco, and dairy products—it forbade them. How could one endure a therapy that banished from the table so many of the things that made eating such a sensuous pleasure? How, for that matter, could cancer be cured by nutrition alone?

Yet Beata *had* been cured—not only of cancer, but of diabetes, frequent migraines, incipient osteoarthritis, and chronic dental abscesses as well. She had even been cured of a thirty year addiction to nicotine. Her cigarette habit had been a problem for us both when we shared a room at one of the weekend conferences we attended.

It was at one such conference that we met when sitting opposite each other at the vegetarian table for lunch. I remember the strong feeling we both had that we had met before. We hadn't, of course; I could not have met someone as distinctive and sophisticated as Beata and forgotten her for an instant. Her poise, her faint but distinctive accent, the way she surveyed me with half-closed eyelids while blowing a stream of smoke toward the ceiling, set her apart from most of our fellow conferees. That day marked the start of our friendship—a friendship that, for me, was enhanced by Beata's knowledge of all the things I was so eager to learn.

By 1980, however, she was coping with cancer, while my struggle with pesticide poisoning had just begun. I don't think either of us fully understood what the other was going through at the time, for there were periods when we scarcely saw each other.

As Beata later confided, "I often felt that we existed in two different kinds of reality." And, in truth, I suppose we did. Beata's reality was clear and focused, grounded in a lifetime of journalism and working toward a practice in psychotherapy for when she retired. My reality was dreamy and formless and wandering all over the place, which drove us both to distraction. Yet there existed between us a curious bond that I don't think either one could have defined.

That night, as my thinning carapace threatened to crumble, Beata's account of her triumph over cancer was just what I needed to get me through the long dark hours until dawn.

I opened her book and read again the inscription she had written on the title page:

For Faye—whose path keeps crossing and touching
mine, with friendship and love,
Beata

I began to read, torn between absorption in her story and envy of her narrative skill, for Beata was a wonderful writer. At the time, she was a features writer for the BBC's World Service and had already published two books. As I read of her struggle with cancer, however, I was reminded of how differently we responded to events of a similar nature. It may even have been our differences that drew us into our singular—if, at times, problematic friendship.

Beata was a transplanted Hungarian and a left-brain Gemini/Scorpio: quick-witted, impatient and intellectual. I was a transplanted American and a right-brain Scorpio/Cancer: slow-witted, absent-minded and self-taught. Yet, as I read of the incurable diagnosis that led her to embark on such a radical journey, I sensed that her story might hold the key to my own darkening dilemma.

If so, it would not be the first time I followed in Beata's footsteps, for she had introduced me to a number of things I would not otherwise have known about or explored—such as the Transpersonal Psychology workshops, which I enjoyed despite the no-show of that sage on the mountaintop. Looking back, I suspect the reason he stood me up was because he knew how unteachable I am by words alone. I seem to need a good kick up the backside to learn anything at all.

When I told Beata I had found my original birth certificate, which gave me not only my parents' names but my hour of birth as well—indispensable for casting a personal horoscope—she took me to one of the finest astrologers in England.

I still have the tape of that reading. Listening to it again, I recalled my amusement when the astrologer said, "Now, your chart shows a strong unconventional side; unusual, eccentric . . . a bit way out," for she could not have been more wrong. There were no conventions I wanted to flout, no rules I wished to defy. On the contrary, I mourned the loss of so many conventions I cherished that were quintessentially English, such as good manners, tolerance, civility, a sly sense of humor and a bemused acceptance of eccentricity. Moreover, I viewed those who strive to be unconventional as absurd.

Reading Beata's book that night, I recalled a discussion we had in the 1980s about my pesticide poisoning. She had suggested I try the Gerson Therapy, but I rejected the idea, reminding her that I had been cancer-free since 1974.

"That doesn't matter," she said. "The therapy is nonspecific—it's not just for cancer."

"Even so," I countered, "how could a vegan regime purge my body of the chemicals it has taken me a lifetime to acquire?"

"Because the therapy detoxifies the body and rebuilds the immune system," she explained with infinite patience. "I see no reason why it shouldn't work for you as it has for me."

Detoxifies the body and rebuilds the immune system—precisely what I knew I needed if health was to be restored. Still, even if this were possible, I wasn't sure I had the strength of will to stick to such a demanding regime. But if not the therapy, what then? I could not go on much longer in my present state.

That night, as I struggled to hold chemical demons at bay, I decided that if Beata's footsteps were leading to Mexico, I would follow them even across the sea. But first, I needed to know more about what the therapy entailed.

I rang her the next day to say how much I was enjoying her book and thanked her for helping me to get through the night.

"Beata," I said, "I'm thinking of doing the Gerson Therapy. When can you come to lunch and give me the shove I need?"

CHAPTER SEVENTEEN

*It is from nature that the disease arises
and from nature comes the cure,
not from the physician.*
—Paracelsus

She arrived looking wonderfully fit and full of energy, her mind as quick and incisive as ever, her tongue only occasionally sharp-edged. As proof of the therapy's success, Beata could not have been bettered. We embraced and after catching up on our separate lives, I got down to the matter at hand.

"I don't know what to do about the chemicals in my system, Beata. I've tried everything I can think of, but nothing has worked. I just become more sensitive to more things and more discouraged. While reading your book, it came to me that since I've run out of options I might as well try the Gerson therapy."

"Good!" she exclaimed, pleased to have gotten through to me at last. "As you know, I've felt for some time that a good detox with hyper-nutrition would be bound to improve your condition, if it doesn't cure it completely."

"What I find off-putting is the prospect of all those juices, not to mention the coffee enemas!"

Beata laughed. "They're really not as bad as they sound. Anyway," she said, with a slight whiff of condescension, "as you don't have cancer, you probably won't be doing the full intensive therapy. I expect you will only have to do the modified diet, with fewer juices and enemas."

The mild put-down should not have rankled, for I knew it was unintended, but it did. Well, dammit, I'd *had* cancer ten years before. I had even given a breast to the disease, which some might think a worse disfigurement than a scar on the shin. But then I realized that Beata was only reflecting the universal view: that cancer is the Queen Bee of diseases—or rather, the Queen C; the one against which all toxic threats are measured and that receives the most funding, with the poorest return on that investment.

Then, too, like most people, Beata had no idea what environmental illness entailed. I thought of the year before, when I was on crutches with my foot in a cast; how eagerly strangers offered to help, how quickly cars came to a halt if they saw me standing on the corner—and how quickly they would have sped on, had their sympathy been sought for the invisible, yet far worse infirmity within. With no lump or bump to display, no fearful label to intone, my predicament inspired derision more often than sympathy.

"As for the vegetable juices," Beata was saying, "you'll need the kind of juicing machine that grinds the vegetables— not a centrifugal one—and also a separate press. The trouble with centrifugal juicers is that they produce an exchange of positive and negative electricity, which destroys the oxidizing enzymes needed to restore the immune system."

"But why so many juices?" I asked. "Isn't it eight or ten a day?"

"Thirteen, actually, at the start."

"Thirteen! Doesn't the body rebel?"

"Not really," she said, with an indulgent smile. "The reason for so many juices is because the depleted body has to be bombarded at short and regular intervals with all the live vitamins, minerals and oxidizing enzymes they contain. It's only in juice form, you see, that the necessary huge amounts can be taken and absorbed."

"And the coffee enemas—why coffee? It seems perverse to be putting it up your backside while forbidding its more pleasurable consumption."

Beata laughed. "It has an altogether different effect when used at the other end," she explained. "The caffeine dilates the bile ducts, thus allowing the liver to release toxic accumulations. It stimulates an enzyme system in the liver, which is able to remove free radicals from the bloodstream. The coffee enema was one of the great German discoveries of the 1920s. Gerson began using them in the 30s and now they're included in many naturopathic therapies."[13]

"But why does the therapy take so long? Eighteen months seems an unconscionable time to have to endure such deprivation."

"Well, Gerson believed that it takes approximately five to six weeks for each liver cell to divide and produce a healthier daughter cell. And for real liver health, perhaps fifteen new generations of increasingly healthier liver cells need to come into being."

"Not a therapy for the fainthearted, then," I observed. Rigorous and restricting, it seemed more than body or spirit could bear: a sentence of eighteen months to two years, at the end of which one might or might not be cured. Yet, if one *could* be cured . . . . After all, it had taken more than two years for my immune system to collapse; more like eighteen.

"You must read Gerson's book," said Beata. "You can get it at the health food store on Baker Street. Skip the clinical bits—they can be heavy going. Just read the easier how-to sections. I'll give you Charlotte's phone number at the Gerson Institute in San Diego.[14] The institute is near the border, about half an hour from the clinic. Tell her you've spoken with me and ask when they can accommodate you.

"Oh," she added, "and you'll need a full-time helper when you return, to make the juices and prepare the organic meals. It's almost impossible to do this on your own, especially when you're having a flare-up."

"A flare-up?"

---

[13] Coffee enemas were included in *Merck's Manual* until 1973.

[14] Charlotte Gerson, Dr. Gerson's daughter, has been carrying on his work since her father's death in 1959.

"A healing reaction," she explained—"I think you Americans call it 'the Herxheimer response'—symptoms get worse, temporarily, as the healing process kicks in and toxins begin to move into the bloodstream. That's when you'll need someone to keep the raw vegetable juices coming, because you'll be too ill to make them yourself."

A daunting prospect indeed, before which I felt myself starting to quail. I wasn't good at long-term commitment, and now that I was committing to do the therapy, the familiar panic set in. Still, if I wanted to get well, I had no choice but to bite the bullet, as Clive would say—or perhaps "bite the carrot" was nearer the mark.

"I'm glad you've decided to take the plunge," said Beata, as we walked to the door. "I'm sure you'll find that it's the right step."

"I hope so," I replied, "because if it isn't . . . ." I left the sentence unfinished, afraid to give voice to its implication.

"And now that you'll be joining the club," added Beata as we embraced, "don't you think we should be seeing a bit more of each other?"

The next day, I went to Baker Street and bought Gerson's book, *A Cancer Therapy: Results of Fifty Cases*. The cover bore an impressive tribute:

I see in Dr. Max Gerson one of the most eminent geniuses in medical history.
Albert Schweitzer

Gerson, I learned, had cured Schweitzer's wife of lung tuberculosis, after conventional treatments failed. Later, he cured Schweitzer of advanced diabetes when he was seventy-five.

Returning home with my purchase, I was conscious of facing a crossroad similar to the one Beata faced three years earlier. The difference was that I knew someone for whom the therapy had worked. Whether it would work for me was far from certain.

I stretched out on the sofa with the book and a bag of potato chips, relishing the guilty pleasure I always felt when reading a book in the daytime—the legacy of a doting stage mother, who, when she saw me with my nose in a book, said, "Shouldn't you be improving yourself, dear, instead of just wasting time?"

I began my delicious waste of time by skipping through the pages at random, reading a sentence here, a paragraph there, until I came upon the following passage:

> Metabolism and immune system are gradually damaged over a long period of time by inadequate nutrition: food grown on a depleted, artificially fertilized soil that does not contain the necessary minerals; food deficient in proteins and potassium, made toxic by chemicals, processed and refined until it contains no live, active nutrients without which health cannot be maintained.

I stopped. The processed and refined chip in my mouth tasted suddenly stale, its chemical crunch a bit less satisfying than before. I turned the bag over and read the ingredients on the back: "Dehydrated, partially hydrogenated, artificial color . . . ." I set the bag aside and read on.

> The malnourished body is then made even more toxic by environmental pollution; impure air and water, chemicals at large everywhere. Eventually, the hidden starvation and the accumulation of toxins combine to cause a breakdown in the body's defense system, so that a tumor can develop.

Gerson wrote this in the 1950s, concerned even then with ecological issues that, today, are still being contested in certain halls of denial. Yet he was not the first to advocate pure food and water as the key to lasting health. In 1809,

113

Richard Lambe, MD, of London, published a treatise on the successful treatment of cancer by a diet of fruits, vegetables and pure water. Like Gerson, Lambe eventually extended his diet to include the treatment of all diseases.

Long before our latter-day health gurus made nutrition fashionable (and profitable), Gerson in Germany, Norman Walker in the U.S. and others, were preaching similar diets for the prevention and cure of degenerative diseases—preaching, moreover, to a deaf and scoffing medical establishment. Not much has changed. Then, as now, one could always tell a pioneer by the arrows in his back.

As Sir Almroth Wright phrased it in his well-known dictum:

Each new idea in medicine has to pass through three stages:

When it is regarded as ridiculous;

When doctors say "It may be possible, but where is the proof?"

When it is finally dismissed by everyone as obvious.

I read the transcript of a talk Gerson gave three years before his death, in which he explained the evolution of his therapy. It began, he said, with his early success with tuberculosis. That led to patients with terminal cancer seeking his help, which in turn brought him an increasing number of hopeless conditions.

"I was forced into that," he observed wryly. "On the one side, the knife of the AMA was at my throat and on my back I had only terminal cases. If I had not saved them, my clinic would have been a death house. I learned that in tuberculosis and in all other degenerative diseases, one must not treat the symptoms. The body—the whole body—has to be treated."

One must not treat the symptoms! The words leapt up at me from the page. Here was a German-Jewish doctor, driven from his country and scorned in mine, saying something that sounded so sensible, yet so radical, it seemed like revelation. I read on avidly, marking the passages that spoke to my condition.

Gerson maintained that most disease is the manifestation of an improperly functioning immune system; that if the body's metabolism can be restored, it will heal itself. All well and good, but his therapy evolved in the 1930s, before the post-war proliferation of chemicals began to spread its poison over the planet. How could carrot juice restore a shattered immune system? How could a vegan diet remove chemicals absorbed from the very fruits and vegetables that I, a long-time vegetarian, had been consuming for years?

On the 23rd of July, I reached Charlotte Gerson on the telephone. Her voice was strong and reassuring, with just the hint of a German accent. I explained that I had cancer in 1974 and asked if she thought the therapy could purge the pesticides from my body.

"It can," she said, "if you haven't had chemotherapy or too many drugs."

"No chemo, fortunately, but far too many tranquillizers and antibiotics over the years. Do you think it could cure my allergies as well?"

"Of course. The process is the same. My father stressed that the therapy is 'nonspecific.' But I cannot promise you a quick cure. You will have to be prepared to stay on the therapy for some time."

"Longer than the eighteen months required for cancer patients?"

"I don't know. We can only judge that when you're here. But there are no quick fixes for the toxic body. It is a slow, hard slog that tests one's endurance to the limit. You should plan to stay at the clinic for at least three weeks," she advised, "because the initial detoxification can produce strong flare-ups, which it would be better to experience under the doctor's supervision."

We fixed my arrival for the 26th of August. That would give me a week to spend with my widowed father in Los Angeles, curtailing the normal four-week pilgrimage I made each summer. It would also give me a chance to see my daughters again. I had missed them since Kate and Amy left England to live in California. Neither girl was given to letter-writing or picking up a phone. I would need those last precious days with them before going into purdah.

There was so much to do before departure the tasks ahead seemed daunting. Yet, from the moment I committed to the therapy, each step fell effortlessly into place—even to finding a Portuguese helper, whose long-time employer had recently died and who could start in September, after taking a month's vacation at home.

With dietary restrictions now only weeks away, I embarked on a manic food binge—sanctioned, I kept telling myself, by a rash of social engagements that exposed me to temptation—and to smoke-filled rooms. This posed a dilemma: my lungs or my social life? At one dinner party, the hosts, who claimed to be spiritually evolved, held forth on the dangers of pollution while puffing clouds of smoke over the proudly prepared organic fare. Their self-delusion was only marginally worse than my own, which continued to balk at connecting the kind of food I was feeding my body with its multiplying symptoms and mounting rebellion.

CHAPTER EIGHTEEN

Swiftly, with nothing spared, I am being dismantled.
—St. John of the Cross

By August, I could no longer remain in the flat after dark. Here, too, there were energies that felt stronger at night—or perhaps I was reacting to some new influence yet to be identified. If the flight to Mexico was not to become an emergency, I would need to find a temporary bolt hole for the remaining nights in London.

I found a small hotel off the Brompton Road and booked a room for the week until departure. I had been in bed but a short time when familiar symptoms alerted me to the presence of an allergen in the room. Wearily, I got up and did a sniff test, but was unable to pin down the source. It might have been organotins—chemicals found in most hotel furnishings, mattresses, and bed linens, which are toxic even in small quantities—or some other odorless chemical impossible to detect.

Whatever the source, I knew I couldn't stay. It was too late to find another hotel and I couldn't return to the flat, so I got dressed and drove aimlessly through the streets of Fulham, fighting discouragement and aching for sleep.

Toward half-past ten a light rain began to fall. Finding myself on Manresa Road, I pulled over to the curb, released the Honda's reclining seat for the first time and attempted to doze. While the rain drummed monotonously down, images flickered in the retina of my mind—scenes of a distant past and a distant me—a time when I took vigor for granted and health was an eternal birthright.

I saw the woman shopper in the lingerie department at Harrods, who told me her skin was so sensitive the only fabric she could tolerate against it was silk. I saw the convention hall in Vermont where I was eating a piece of carrot cake, when a caftan with beads glided past me, chiding sweetly, "Dead food!" And I saw the roadside spit in a Turkish village, where friends who sampled the meat came down with food poisoning, which I escaped.

The first hint of dawn crept through the windows. Stiff and unrefreshed, I returned the car's seat to its vertical position and drove home to shower and change. Then I rang Clive to tell him of my decision. He already knew about the therapy—as much as he cared to know—so my news did not come as a complete surprise.

"I know now, Clive, that unless I can get these chemicals out of my system, I'll be unable to live on this planet, so this is my last hope."

"Well, my dear," he said, in a voice much warmer than usual, "I think you've made the right decision." I suspected the warmth in his voice owed less to hope for my recovery than to relief at getting me off his back.

Later that morning, I returned to the hotel to let the manager know I would not be keeping the room. He didn't mind; the tourist season was at its height.

"Oh, by the way," I added, "have you by any chance fumigated the beds recently?" He looked faintly alarmed, as though anticipating a bedbug complaint.

"No, but we do that once a year. They were fumigated in January. Why?"

"Oh. Then perhaps that explains it."

"Explains what?"

"Well, you see . . . I'm chemically sensitive, and I may have been affected by a residue of the fumigant, whatever it was."

"But you couldn't have been," he said, laughing. "That was seven months ago!"

"Oh, yes . . . of course," I said, and let it go at that.

I found a room as a paying guest in the flat of a woman who lived across the square. A quick dowse of the bed proved it to be safe, although two of the energy lines that ran through my flat ran elsewhere through hers as well. This was not surprising, for these energies extend indefinitely—how far we do not know. At least, I hoped, I might get some sleep for the remaining nights in London.

Lying awake in a strange bed so near to my own, I tried not to think what would happen if I returned from Mexico more sensitive than when I left; if I could never again live in my flat—or anywhere else, for that matter, except perhaps on a desert island. Yet I *had* to be in my home to do the therapy. I couldn't decamp each night with a 68-pound juicing machine, a bag of carrots and a Portuguese helper.

Two days before departure, I rang Beata.

"Just as a precaution, Beata—in case the Portuguese lady lets me down—do you know anyone here who might be able to help with the juices for a week or two when I return?"

"There's a man here who gets people started on the therapy," she said, "but with so many cancer patients needing help, I'm sure you'll agree their need takes priority." Priority? Who but the most desperate sufferer would even consider embarking on such a Draconian regime? "You should start the coffee enemas immediately," Beata advised. "You'll need a quart of the coffee liquid and be sure to lie on your right side. The reason for this is so the coffee will turn the corner of the colon from the descending to the transverse colon at the splenic flexure."

The body's internal infrastructure being a total mystery to me, the thought of all those densely packed, convoluted, descending and transverse tubes was distinctly worrying. I only hoped Max Gerson knew what he was about when he added this coffee lark to his therapy.

119

Having been spared enemas as a child I had no hang-ups about them, so to speak, but neither did I know quite how to go about the procedure. Beata explained how to make the coffee solution, but when I asked her what to do after that—a silly question, admittedly—her mirth was so humiliating ("Surely you have the wit to figure it out for yourself, read Gerson's book,") I felt too stupid to press her further.

I flipped through the book, but Gerson must have assumed most people knew the drill. I bought an enema bag and prepared the brew, then wondered at what height the thing should be hung. The bathroom doorknob looked too low, and with no visible object of medium height that could serve as a hook, I ended up suspending the bag from a four-foot standing lamp in the study. This precipitated such an inrush—and outrush of liquid, the whole enterprise ended in disaster and stomach cramps.

Beata might have warned me! I thought crossly, as I tidied up the floor.

On the 17th of August, I flew to Los Angeles, fighting my usual in-flight headache while spurning the painkillers that would have added to the chemicals I was going to Mexico to shed. In Los Angeles, I stayed with my father and spent a happy week with my daughters, wondering when I would see them again. I called the Gerson Institute on the 26th to confirm my arrival, a friend having offered to drive me to San Diego.

"If you can be here by half-past eight in the morning," said the coordinator, "Charlotte will drive you to the clinic herself, since it's one of her visiting days. By the way," he added, "will you have trouble negotiating the stairs?"

I explained that my problem was pesticide poisoning, not cancer, and that it manifested primarily as multiple allergies.

"Oh, allergies can take much longer to cure than cancer," he said. "Once your immune system has been repaired, you may have to remain on a modified version of the therapy for some years."

Ah, well, I thought, so much for priorities.

CHAPTER NINETEEN

What we eat has changed more in the last
forty years than in the previous 40,000.
—Eric Schlosser

I was standing outside the Gerson Institute on the morning of the 26th, when a car drove up and a tall grey-haired
woman of imposing stature stepped out.

"You must be Faye," she said, advancing with out-
stretched hand. "Hello, I'm Charlotte Gerson."

She was much as I had imagined she would be: the quick
step, the commanding presence, and the sense of coiled
energy that seems to inhabit those who devote their lives to a
holy purpose. I put my suitcase, typewriter, and portable air
purifier in the back seat of her car and we set off for the
Mexican border seven miles away. Charlotte asked after
Beata, whose glowing health and warmest greetings I was
pleased to convey.

"About your symptoms," she said. "I understand they
manifest primarily as allergies?"

Uncertain as to how she would respond to their more
esoteric manifestations, I framed my answer with care.

"The main problem is pesticide poisoning," I began,
"which has weakened my immune system in a way that has
made me sensitive to some peculiar things."

"Such as?"

I described my experience with earth energies and the
polluted stream, explaining how the latter led inadvertently
to my discovery of water divining. I needn't have feared her

reaction. Dowsing has a long and respected history in Germany, and Charlotte was as knowledgeable about the arcane as she was about cancer.

Shortly after we crossed the border, I noticed a marked change in the landscape. The neatly groomed houses surrounded by greenery gave way to a scene of dust and disrepair. Clusters of *favelas* sprawled on a hillside, their makeshift materials festooned with colorful washing lines— the garlands of poverty. Clapped-out American cars bumped along the pockmarked road, some with dented fenders and one with a bumper hanging half off.

My interest in the scenery, however, was only intermittent, for I was more interested in what Charlotte was saying. I had asked her why the clinic was in Mexico instead of California.

"It's in Mexico," she explained, "because it's against the law in California to treat cancer by any means other than surgery, radiation, or drugs, even though nutrition is safe and has no side effects."

"But how was such a law passed?" I asked. "In whose interest could it have been?"

"The pharmaceutical companies, of course," she replied. "They have powerful lobbies in every state and the American Medical Association is in their pocket. Its journal relies heavily on their advertising revenue, so the chemical companies got our lawmakers to rule that to treat cancer you can only slash, burn, or poison. But then you know this yourself, don't you?" she added, referring to the mastectomy I mentioned on the telephone.

"But wasn't the purpose of the law to protect the gullible from quacks?"

"Well, of course there are quacks in every profession. But what about all the patients who die after having surgery and radiation, or those who suffer terrible side effects from chemotherapy and *still* die in the end? Ninety-five percent of the patients we see here are terminal cases," said Charlotte. "They come to us *after* having been treated by orthodox doctors—who, by the way, have taken a fortune from them as well, yet, nobody calls those doctors quacks."

I glanced at the handsome woman sitting beside me; this bucker of the Establishment, this latter-day St. Joan who was fighting the same battles her father fought forty years earlier against an entrenched monopoly—and lost. It was sobering to reflect that if Jesus returned tomorrow and fetched up in this land of the free, he could be arrested for practicing medicine without a license. And if he tried to raise the dead without drugs he could be thrown in jail.

Where were the civil liberties groups when the laws curtailing our freedom of medical choice were being enacted?

"Well, here we are," said Charlotte, swinging the car through a broad gate and into the forecourt of La Gloria Hospital. Compared to the arid landscape through which we had passed, La Gloria appeared an oasis, with well-kept grounds and a reassuring aspect of order.

We stopped in front of two long, low, single-story buildings, beyond which I saw a flight of steps that led up a sloping hill to a larger two-story structure. "That's the main building," said Charlotte. "This is the annex and the administration building." She led me into the office to register and receive an information folder. A large portrait of Dr. Gerson looked down on us from the wall, his expression sober, the keen blue eyes intelligent, observing. There was a look of stubbornness about him, but of kindliness as well.

I had asked Charlotte if I could have a quiet room, since I hoped to do some work while there.

"Follow me," she said and led me through a corridor of the annex to a room at the very end. "Will this be quiet enough for you?" she inquired, opening the door to invite my inspection.

"It will be perfect," I said, having noticed the neighboring room appeared to be unoccupied.

Charlotte smiled. "You might like to know that this was Beata's room when she was here." I laughed with delight.

Not only was I following in Beata's footsteps—like an aging Goldilocks, I was sleeping in her bed as well.

"You'll find distilled water in the cooler outside the door," said Charlotte. "It's the only kind we use here."

She left me to unpack and I surveyed my surroundings. They were those of any modest motel, save for the plastic-covered bench at the foot of the bed, which had an iron pole attached at one end with a double hook at the top for the enema bucket. Suspended from the ceiling was a curtain that could be drawn around the bench for privacy. Noting the carafe of coffee being kept warm on a hot plate beside the bed, I wondered how many caffeine addicts had broken the "no coffee by mouth" rule and secretly quaffed the odd cup.

Beata had warned that the facilities at La Gloria were fairly primitive, but that didn't bother me.[15] What did concern me were the many synthetic fabrics in the room: the PVC-covered bench, the polyester sheets and pillowcases—even a soft, plastic cover on the toilet seat! And already, my nose was recoiling from the strong disinfectant in the bathroom.

I began to unpack, removing the rod and color wheel I'd brought so I could check the room for energy lines. Happily, it dowsed quiet. Just then, the small desk arrived that Charlotte had kindly arranged for me to borrow. It took up most of the space in the room, but accommodated my electronic typewriter, diary and supplies.

I was hanging up my clothes when I heard a knock at the open door and turned to see a short, grey-haired woman in a white coat standing in the doorway.

"Good morning," she said in a soft Spanish accent. "I am Dr. Melendez, the doctor assigned to your case."

Her round, smiling face was a welcome change from some of the toffee-nosed doctors I had encountered in London. Dr. Melendez reviewed my medical history and was doing the preliminary blood tests, when a young woman

---

[15] The conditions at La Gloria in 1985 bear no relation to the present Gerson clinic in Baja, Mexico.

from the kitchen appeared with my first glass of carrot and apple juice.

"Patients are put on the therapy as soon as they arrive," Dr. Melendez explained. Moments later, another girl delivered a plate of fruit and three thermoses. "One thermos contains peppermint tea, one, chamomile tea, and the third has oat gruel," said Dr. Melendez. "You should drink and eat as much of these as possible throughout the day."

I was savoring the taste of the organic carrot juice—so much sweeter than the commercial variety—when I noticed the fruit plate was tightly covered with Saran wrap, its plasticizers leaching into the organic produce. I drew Dr. Melendez's attention to this and explained my concern. She looked surprised.

"I'll have to tell them about that," she said, but if she did, nothing was done about it while I was there.

Shortly after she left, a pretty young nurse, Lulu, came to show me how to take an enema. Dimpled and smiling, she chattered away in Spanish while explaining with hand gestures the correct height for the bucket, which I had finally figured out for myself.

Cheerful Lulu was followed by an older nurse who gave the daily injections of crude liver extract with vitamin B_{12}. "You will be administering these to yourself when you return home," she said. Her perfume was so strong I could hardly breathe while she was in the room. How on earth was I going to detoxify in a place so indifferent to environmental hazards?

By lunchtime, I had tasted the green leaf juice in addition to the carrot and apple. The former, a combination of vegetables chosen for their high potassium content, consisted of romaine lettuce, Swiss chard, green pepper, red cabbage, leafy beet tops (but not beets), and apple. I had also tried the carrot and raw liver juice, which tasted like soap.[16] Patients

---

[16] The liver juice was eliminated in 1989, when it was no longer possible to find young calves' livers uncontaminated by helicobacter.

had to down three of these revolting mixtures each day. Ah, well, I thought, at least if I die, I'll die with a healthy liver.

On entering the dining hall for lunch, I was surprised at the air of cheerfulness in the room. Had I not known these were cancer patients, I would have taken them to be a group of friendly tourists on holiday. Counter to what the medical establishment would have us believe, none of the patients I met had "spurned the chance of a cure by choosing the alternative path first," to quote a non-practicing radio doctor. Each had exhausted the conventional route *before* coming to Mexico as a last resort. Those at my table had undergone surgery, chemotherapy and radiation, and still their cancers returned.

Tales of medical mismanagement abounded, some so harrowing they beggared belief. A young farmer from the Midwest, Randy, whose stomach was badly distended with leukemia, told me his story.

"One doctor put me on Myloran without discussing the side effects," he said. "He didn't even ask me to sign the required release form, which included that I understood the risks involved. After taking the damn thing for two days, I felt worse than I did from all the drugs I'd ever taken before—and that includes the hard stuff. I was puking and had a jackhammer headache that wouldn't go away, so I stopped taking it and flushed the rest down the toilet.

"But then I got curious and looked it up in the PDR,[17] and guess what I found: two columns devoted to Myloran's side effects, one of which said it could cause *melanoma*. And *this*," he snorted, "was being given to someone who had leukemia! Not only that, it had been listed as an experimental drug for forty years!"

Listening to Randy's story, I didn't know whether to weep or to rage. Had his oncologist been an alternative practitioner, he would have been hauled before a medical board and struck off for malpractice.

---

[17] *Physicians Desk Reference.*

"And I'll bet you didn't know that no scientific double-blind studies have ever been done on chemotherapy drugs, either," he added.

"But why does your Food and Drug Administration *allow* such dangerous drugs to exist?" asked Tina, a pediatrician from England who'd had a colostomy and now had cancer of the liver.

"Because they have a revolving door with the pharmaceutical companies," said Randy's brother, who was there as his caregiver. "Their officers land cushy jobs with the drug companies when they leave the government, so they spend our tax dollars trying to put alternative therapies out of business."

"I've often wondered," mused Tina, "if my original cancer could have been caused by an exposure to insecticides I had about five years before my diagnosis."

"I believe I can answer that," I said, venturing to join the discussion. "Five years is about the time it takes for cancer to develop after a severe chemical exposure. The reason I know this," I added, flashing my badge of belonging, "is because I had breast cancer and my immune system began to collapse from pesticide poisoning about five years before it was diagnosed."

A schoolteacher from Australia, Hal, spoke up, saying that he, too, had had a colostomy.

"I now have cancer of the rectum," he said. "When my doctor told me my condition was terminal, I decided to come here, although it's probably too late for me to expect a miracle."

"I'll show you a miracle," said Morris, an affable Canadian in his 70's and the senior member of the group. He stood up, placed a foot on the chair and pulled his trouser leg up to the knee to display a slightly discolored shin. "I've had a gangrenous skin condition on both legs for thirty years," he boasted, "and it's almost gone since I started the therapy six months ago. See?" He added that his diabetes and prostate cancer were healing nicely as well. Morris, I learned, was the clinic's longest-staying resident—not because he needed to stay, but because he had fallen in love with Mexico and gone native in a senior citizen sort of way, studying Spanish and attending the local celebrations.

An American woman, Pearl, whose elderly husband was the patient, had clearly been itching to speak. Thin and angular, with kohl-smudged eyes and frizzy bleached hair that bunched over her forehead like a Poodle's, she clinked and winked with silver jewelry, large knuckle-dusters on every finger.

"Harry's prostate cancer came back after chemo, too," said Pearl. "When he told his doctor he was going to come down here, the doc had a fit and tried to talk us out of it, but I told him what he could do with his chemo!"

With her raucous voice and quenchless energy, Pearl brought a liveliness to our table that was missing in her wizened spouse, to whose emaciated arm she clung with a quite unnecessary possessiveness.

And then there was Nora, whose husband, David, had pancreatic cancer that returned after chemo and had metastasized to his bones. To this quiet, middle-aged couple from Montana I felt instantly attuned, so I was saddened to learn they were near the end of their stay and would be leaving in a few days.

The food at La Gloria was organic, vegetarian, and delicious, with a wide variety of dishes to choose from. Two items were to be eaten twice a day: the "Hippocrates" soup—a blend of vegetables chosen for their cleansing effect on the kidneys—and a baked potato. A bottle of flaxseed oil stood on each table with a dish of peeled garlic cloves, flanked by a press. Any therapy that *urged* you to eat garlic, I reckoned, couldn't be wrong.

No bread or dairy products were allowed for the first six weeks. ("The Gerson patient does not fill up on bread," read a stern fiat in the primer.) We were encouraged, however, to eat and drink as much of the permitted foods as possible. My only complaint at the end of two weeks was that there was so much food, I would have welcomed a day of fast.

Each patient received a sectioned pillbox containing the supplements we were to take in a certain order and at certain times during the day. These included niacin, thyroid, and pancreatin tablets, with Acidoll capsules (hydrochloric acid) to aid digestion. Fortunately, we were also given a printed schedule to follow. The juices were delivered hourly to our rooms. Liquid potassium compound was added to every carrot juice, with a drop of Lugol's solution (iodine) added six times a day.

Plunged into a regime that ignored the concept of food rotation and flooded the system with the same vegetables day after day, I wondered how my body would respond to this radical change of direction. Halfway through lunch, my face, arms and bottom broke out in red, stinging splotches, like an angry heat rash.

"Don't worry," said Nora, who was sitting next to me. "It's the niacin flush. It goes away after twenty minutes or so." And so it did.

"How soon do you think I'll have a flare-up?" I asked.

"I can't really say," she replied, "because it's different with each person, but I should think within a few days or a week."

Nora, who could see I needed looking after, reminded me after lunch that it was time for my first "coffee break," the Gerson euphemism for enema time.

"Be sure to hang the sign with the cup of coffee on the door," she reminded me. "That way, if it's time for a juice, they'll know to leave the glass outside your room. They put a cover on it to preserve the precious enzymes, because they deteriorate rapidly."

With so many things to learn, I decided to make a list of the questions I wanted to ask Charlotte when she stopped by later on her postprandial visit to the patients' rooms.

"Don't four coffee enemas a day destroy the lining of the colon?" I began, after switching on the tape recorder Beata advised me to bring ("Your conversations with Charlotte will be important morale boosters when you return to England.")

"Not at all," she said. "You see, to initiate healing, you must detoxify the body, especially the liver-bile system. The caffeine was found to dilate the bile ducts and stimulate discharge of accumulated toxins. The fruit and freshly pressed raw vegetable juices stimulate the kidneys to detoxify the body. Being rich in minerals, enzymes, and vitamins, they start the process of returning these substances to the depleted organs."

"But couldn't this be done more easily by taking capsules with the requisite vits and mins?"

"No," said Charlotte, firmly. "You see, it's not the vitamin A in the carrots that is beneficial, as most people think; it's the *natural* beta-carotene that activates the immune response. A severely toxic and damaged system is unable to absorb and utilize concentrated preparations. Such pills have a tendency to irritate a terminal patient further and cause him to lose more of his own already depleted reserves."

"By the way," I said, thinking longingly of potato chips, "why is salt forbidden on the diet?"

"Because sodium is an enzyme inhibitor," Charlotte explained. "In nature, all foods grow with the proportion of potassium to sodium that the body needs, sometimes as much as a thousand times more potassium than sodium. When foods are processed, they're cooked in such a way that the potassium is lost. Thus, the average diet is heavily unbalanced, with too much salt."

"Which contributes to high blood pressure?"

"High blood pressure returns to normal in five days on the therapy."

I showed Charlotte the antigen vaccines Jean advised me to keep taking.

"Is there a freezer where I could store these while I'm here?" I asked.

Charlotte eyed the vials warily. "You can take those if you wish," she said, "but I don't think you'll need them after the therapy gets underway. We don't have a freezer here because all the food is fresh. The nurses have a refrigerator with a small freezing compartment in their quarters, which I'm sure they'd let you use. How many antigens do you have?"

"About fifty, ten in each vial."

Charlotte reached for one and read the ingredients on the label.

"Personally," she said, handing it back to me, "I don't feel good about injecting chemicals into the body, no matter how diluted they are."

"The antigens did help at first," I said, "but then, for some reason, I seemed to reach a plateau and they stopped working."

"Precisely; because desensitizing vaccines are still just treating the symptoms and not the disease. They desensitize the body, but do not rebuild its capacity to heal itself, nor do they detoxify. And, as my father said, 'Without detoxification, you cannot heal.'"

Impressed by the forcefulness of her manner and the logic of her argument, I decided to forego the antigens while at the clinic.

I was in mid-enema the next morning, bare backside to the door, when I heard a knock and before I could answer, a young man in a white coat entered.

"Good morning!" he said, in a cheery American voice. "My name's John. I'm an assistant here. I've brought you your supplements for the day."

He placed the box on the desk, before turning to address me in a matey manner. "So, how're you doin'?"

"Um . . . fine," I lied, stiff with embarrassment.

"Great! Well, see you tomorrow then," he said, and was gone.

Tomorrow, I vowed, that curtain will be drawn around the bench. La Gloria could be an unsettling place for the intensely private person.

Beata must have hated it.

CHAPTER TWENTY

The body is not built wrongly;
it is being used wrongly.
—Surgeon-Captain T.L. Cleave

"It looks as though Hal is having a setback," said Morris the next morning, noting Hal's absence at the breakfast table. Nora and David were missing too.

"I'm worried about him," said Tina. "He hasn't been doing at all well and he's so alone here. I think we should look in on him, Morris, don't you?"

Tina, whose English reserve bordered on coolness, appeared to have a soft spot for Hal, perhaps because of their mutual colostomies or perhaps because they were both Brits. Turning to me, she said, "Won't you come with us?"

I was about to decline, but checked the inclination for fear of appearing stand-offish. Following them into the annex, I discovered that Hal's room was just a few doors down from mine. We found him propped up in bed, looking like death and surrounded by the familiar emblems of the sickroom: damp towels on the floor, clothes strewn about, an open Bible on the nightstand and next to it, an untouched glass of carrot juice.

On seeing us, Hal's face brightened. "I've been running a fever since lunch yesterday," he said in a hoarse whisper. "Can't eat anything . . . the juices . . . can't get them down."

While Tina and Morris chatted with Hal, their visit bringing him evident pleasure, I stood by feeling shy and irrelevant, like the new girl at school invited to join an established clique.

"Oh dear," said Tina, glancing at her watch, "it's time for my coffee break, Hal. I'm in the upper building, so I'll have to make tracks if I'm not to fall behind schedule."

"Me, too," said Morris. "If we don't see you at breakfast tomorrow, Hal, we'll check up on you again, okay?"

I said good-bye and moved to join them, but Hal said, "Please don't go—unless you have to. It's so good to have company for a change."

I hesitated, wanting to leave, but he looked so ill and so lonely I didn't have the heart to refuse. Shifting his bathrobe from the only chair to the table, I drew the chair up to his bed, hoping that Hal would do most of the talking.

"Tell me about yourself, Hal," I said, smiling encouragingly. "You're a teacher, I believe. What do you teach?"

"I was a chemistry teacher," he said, and went on to tell me about his family, his long fight with cancer and his fear the disease had progressed beyond all hope of reversal. At one point he made a sudden grimace and his voice faltered. Beads of sweat appeared on his forehead and without thinking, I stretched out my hand to feel his brow. Hal closed his eyes, covered my hand with his and murmured, "Oh, that feels good . . . a cool hand on my forehead."

I smiled to myself. My hands were always cold; Reynaud's disease, the doctors said. Well—at least the condition could serve some useful purpose.

We sat in silence for a while, thinking our separate thoughts, neither of us feeling the need to speak. I noted the damp patches on his pillow and the passages heavily underscored in red in the open Bible. I, too, when a young and ardent Christian Scientist, underlined my favorite Bible passages, only I did so in blue. Had someone told me then that I would be sitting in a cancer clinic one day, feeling as close to God with the terminally ill as I ever felt in church, I would have disbelieved them.

My mind was thus wandering, when I felt a queasiness in my stomach. Surely this couldn't be a flare-up so soon, yet I never had stomach trouble. I was wondering what could be causing it, when something an astrologer told me years ago returned to mind:

"Now you must never enter the nursing profession," she warned. "You're too vulnerable, like an emotional sponge. You absorb other people's problems and can't help being affected by them—physically as well as emotionally."

At the time her words struck me as hugely funny, for I was being affected by almost everything in the environment. Now, however, I wondered if my hand could be absorbing Hal's symptoms—the way it seemed to absorb the Dacron that day at the clinic. Whatever the cause, I knew I couldn't stay.

"Hal," I said, after a suitable interval, "I'm afraid I must go now—it's coffee break time. But, if you like, I can stop by again on my way to dinner."

"Please do," he whispered—adding, with a feeble smile, "for another laying on of hands?"

The heat in my room was oppressive. Exhausted, I fell onto the bed, hoping the nausea would pass. Only then did I remember my right foot; it was swollen when I got up that morning, but in my preoccupation with Hal I had forgotten about it. Now, I realized the edema had reached my ankle.

A short time later, Dr. Melendez came in. Seeing my prostrate form on the bed, she smiled.

"Your fatigue is caused by the potassium added to the juices," she explained. "The body is not accustomed to the sudden correction of pH imbalance, the change from an acidic to an alkaline state."

Then that could explain the queasiness, I thought, relieved.

"May I skip a couple of juices today?" I pleaded, fearing I might not keep them down.

"No," she said, firmly. "It is important to adhere to the therapy if you possibly can. One cannot eliminate the more difficult parts. Those who have tried to do this did not heal well." I sighed and drew her attention to my swollen foot.

"You must have had an injury to that foot at some time," she observed, "because the swelling is a sign the healing reaction has begun. The allergic inflammation is vital to the healing process."

Injury to my foot? Then I remembered: Baer... the swollen calf... the forgotten suture.

Dr. Melendez left to continue her rounds and I fell asleep. When I woke, I found I had slept through lunch and two juices, both of which, covered, were waiting outside my door, their enzymes long since evaporated.

Recalling that Norman Frye, co-director of the institute, was giving a talk that afternoon, I forced myself to get up. ("You will find the lectures wonderfully educational," said Beata, "especially Charlotte's.")

Frye was already speaking when I reached the room, so I slipped into a seat at the back. A neat, amiable man in his fifties, with sandy hair and moustache, he was talking about a young eight year-old patient, a Hungarian boy, Tamas, who was cured of Ewing's sarcoma.

"This is a diffuse endothelial myeloma that forms tumors on long bones, for which the medical prognosis is very poor," Frye explained. "The boy was treated with chemotherapy prior to coming to Mexico, but the cancer spread from his pelvis into the soft tissues. He was pale and thin and had lost his hair when he came to us, but he was surprisingly well-disciplined and willing to eat the unsalted vegetarian food and drink the juices. He continued the regime when he returned home and now, after two years, he's a strong and healthy lad of ten.

"What makes his recovery even more dramatic," Frye added, "is that he was one of seven children with Ewing's sarcoma who were being treated with chemotherapy in the same Hungarian hospital. Unfortunately, the other six boys died."

Later, I learned it was Beata who met the mothers of the children while on a visit to Hungary and urged them to try the therapy. Only Tamas's mother decided to risk the nutritional path.

Intrigued by the story, and noting that patients were free to interrupt, I raised my hand and asked, "How does a child so young get cancer?"

For a moment, Frye looked discomposed. "Well," he said, "we won't go into that now."

His response surprised me. Why not go into it now? Surely we need to know why the incidence of cancer in children is rising. Did the mother smoke while pregnant? Was she exposed to chemicals? Or did she do drugs? Fifty years ago, cancer in children was almost unheard of. Yet even in 1962, Rachel Carson observed:

> A quarter-century ago, cancer in children was considered a medical rarity. *Today, more American school children die of cancer than from any other disease.* (Italics hers.)

My query went unanswered, for Frye had moved on and was now addressing the subject of flare-ups.

"These can occur at any time" he said, "within days or weeks of starting the therapy. They are the body's vigorous attempts to detoxify and heal itself and the first are usually the worst. Gradually, they'll become shorter and milder, until they disappear altogether. But the symptoms can be nasty," he warned. "Old scars and wounds may turn red, arthritic joints may grow more inflamed and swollen, and headaches, weakness and so forth may become worse for a while. Old drug deposits, too—whether from aspirin or LSD—when being flushed from the body fat into the bloodstream, can produce a stronger effect than when they were being absorbed over a period of time.

"In sum," he concluded, "you are being asked to take charge of your own medical care, but you are being given nature's tools with which to do the job. Unfortunately, many are unable or unwilling to make the required changes in their lives. Difficult though the days ahead may be, I urge you not to panic when flare-ups occur for they are signs the immune system is beginning to reactivate its defenses."

By the end of the lecture the nausea had gone. I was still desperately tired, however, so I returned to my room and slept until dinnertime. On the way to the dining hall, I looked in on Hal. He was no better, so I sat with him for a bit, thinking how lonely he must be—so far from home and in pain, with no loved ones near to comfort him. How I wished my hand could *heal* sickness, instead of absorb it.

My thoughts were running along this line, when that inner voice I was learning to trust whispered: *He's not going to make it. It's too late; he needs hospice care.* But hospice was for those who have accepted death. Hal was grasping this last desperate chance for life. A great sadness came over me then, which I could not shake off for the rest of the evening.

CHAPTER TWENTY-ONE

We are in a vast riddle, all of us – dependence
on a strength that is inimical to life.
—E.B. White

At dinner that evening, I sat next to a woman who told me she was there as the caregiver for her friend, Marie, who had breast cancer.

"When the doctors found the cancer had spread," she said, "they removed some lymph nodes from under her arm, which caused severe lymphedema. I think the procedure is called an 'axillary node dissection.' When we arrived here ten days ago, Marie's arm was so swollen it stuck out at a right angle to her body. She couldn't dress herself or comb her hair, which is why we've been having our meals brought to the room. The swelling has almost gone now and some dark stuff has started to come out on her breast around the nipple. The doctor says it's the dead cancer cells exiting through her pores."

This was so hard to believe I asked if I could meet her friend after dinner.

Marie was sitting up in bed, reading, when we arrived. A good-natured woman in her fifties, she responded willingly to my questions. To show me how swollen her arm was when she arrived, she held it straight out to the side, like a cop directing traffic.

"See?" she said, letting the arm fall. "Now the swelling is gone and I can even comb my hair. And look at this," she added, drawing the top of her robe to one side to reveal her breast and the dark crusts around the nipple. "The dead cancer cells are coming out through my skin."

Had I not witnessed this, I'm not sure I would have believed it. Yet I was reading a book by an earlier Gerson patient, Jaquie Davison, who, like Beata, had been cured of melanoma. She, too, described the dead cancer cells exiting through her pores, only hers came out through the soles of her feet.

Reflecting on Marie as I walked back to my room, I thought how different this approach was from that of the rotary diet. Here, they cured cancer with juices of remorseless repetition, so in theory I should be getting worse. Yet the edema in my foot had subsided, my hair had regained some of its curl, and if there were energy lines at the clinic I was scarcely aware of them. If only I had known about the therapy when I had breast cancer.

On entering my room I found two small paper cups on the desk, one containing brown sugar, the other castor oil. I knew they were for the castor oil enema in the morning, but wasn't sure when to take it or how, so I rang the nurse's office. A woman answered in Spanish.

"Habla Ingles?" I asked, in my high school Spanish.

"Si, si," said the voice and hung up.

Assuming someone would come to the room or ring back, I waited. And waited. When forty minutes passed, I gave up and went to bed. Thank goodness it wasn't an emergency, I thought. This mañana way of life takes some getting used to.

When John arrived at six the next morning (my coffee break postponed until after his visit), I asked, "What am I supposed to do with the castor oil?"

"You should have taken it at five this morning, along with the coffee in the thermos. Didn't they bring you any?"

"No."

"I'll have them send you some. The cup contains two tablespoons of castor oil. If you knock it back with the coffee, you won't taste a thing. Your regular enema is taken an hour later. Four hours after that, you do the castor oil enema. That's what the extra bucket is for."

I had no problem downing the castor oil, but the enema five hours later was a misery to administer. To enable the viscous liquid to slide down the hose, it had to be mixed with water and castile soap and stirred constantly with a wooden spoon until the bucket was drained. The result—not to put too fine a point on it—was like giving birth to a battleship. Trust a Teuton, I thought, albeit a Jewish one, to find a cure that rapes the colon.

By contrast, I quite liked the coffee enemas, for apart from the feeling of cleanliness that resulted, they promised fifteen minutes of quiet reading time. Much of my education in allergy, nutrition, the environment, and the spiritual subjects I was exploring, occurred while I was lying on a bench in Mexico with my nose stuck in a book and a hose stuck up my bottom.

But why do enemas receive such a bad press? I wondered. In an age when no aspect of sex is any longer taboo, nor any orifice a mystery; when pornography is available at the click of a mouse and we've even had a president who taught sixth graders the meaning of oral sex, it does seem a bit prissy to go all squeamish at the thought of cleansing the colon.

Charlotte was waiting in my room when I returned after lunch on the 29th. I switched on the tape recorder and we began our conversation. At one point, thinking of Hal, I asked if she knew what the failure rate was for the therapy.

"Well, you must realize," she said, "that almost all the patients we see here have metastasized cancers no longer treatable by orthodox methods, so of course there are failures. We have a high dropout rate as well. Not everyone has the self-discipline to stick with the therapy when the going gets rough. Some patients drop out after a few months, because they can't cope with the flare-ups."

They had my sympathy, but I would not be one of them. When I committed to the regime, I vowed that if it failed the fault would not be mine.

"But to answer your question," Charlotte continued. "As far as we can tell, we have a twenty to thirty percent success rate."[18]

Small by conventional standards, perhaps, but if the alternative was certain death? I put to Charlotte the same question I put to Norman Frye the day before.

"Tell me, Charlotte, why do *you* think children are getting cancer at a younger and younger age? After all, they aren't old enough to have acquired much in the way of a toxic burden."

"Well, one of the main problems is pesticides," she said, "but there are other reasons as well. Fluoride in the water is one, but also immunization at six weeks when they do the DPT.[19] The dangers of this have been thoroughly documented in a number of studies—all, of course, ignored by the immunization lobbies."

I thought of two couples I knew whose sons, normal at birth, had become brain-damaged after vaccination. One boy was now autistic, while the other was mentally retarded and in a wheelchair. Both had older sisters who were unaffected by the same vaccines. Perhaps the male immune system is weaker at birth than the female, I speculated. All the same, I could not agree with Charlotte that all immunizations are bad. After all, polio had been virtually eradicated with the Salk vaccine. Unwilling to challenge her on the subject, however, and thinking of my daughters' vaccinations, I said,

"I had no idea immunization was unsafe."

"You cannot believe how dangerous it is," said Charlotte. "The earlier it is done the worse, because the immune system is not yet developed at that age. We saw such a case here some time ago. A young mother came as a companion to her father, who had cancer. Because she was nursing, she brought her baby along. But the baby, who was three months old, arrived in a state of respiratory distress.

---

[18] The success rate has greatly increased since 1985.

[19] Diphtheria, pertussis, and tetanus.

"When it was six weeks old the doctor said, 'She's doing so well we can start the DPT shot.' Shortly afterward, the child had trouble breathing, and if you can't breathe, you can't nurse. So the mother—worried, but not suspecting the connection, went back to the doctor, who gave the child some drugs. And it got worse. So what do you do if drugs make a child worse? You give it *more* drugs, right?" she said, her voice dripping with sarcasm. "That's what the doctor did and *still* the child grew worse. She cried at night and couldn't sleep or nurse. This was the state she was in when they arrived here.

"Now, we didn't touch the child," said Charlotte. "We *never* treat a baby. But since this mother was nursing, we treated her. We put her on a lot of vitamin C and carrot juice, with potassium and enemas, and in three days the baby was fine."

"That's the most powerful argument I've heard for breast feeding—and for pure nutrition."

"Well, the therapy is not just a cure for cancer," she reminded me, "or for this or that disease. By restoring and strengthening the *whole* immune system, it restores the body's ability to cure itself."

But would this work for a chemically poisoned body? I wondered.

"Ah, well," said Charlotte, rising, "I have more patients to see, so I'd better be on my way."

I switched off the recorder and rose to accompany her. At the door she paused, turned, and said, with an air of infinite sadness, "What a world we live in, eh?" Then she was gone, her swift, determined footsteps echoing down the corridor.

For some moments after she left I sat thinking about her; her dedication, her courage, and the vast amount of knowledge she acquired during the years she worked at her father's side. I thought of her long struggle to keep his therapy alive and the encouragement she gave to each and every patient in the clinic, week after week, year after year.

And I decided that in my pantheon of saints, Charlotte Gerson stood very near the top.

CHAPTER TWENTY-TWO

*In science the credit goes to the man who
convinces the world, not to the man to
whom the idea first occurs.*
—Sir William Osler

I had been reading Jaquie Davison's book, *Cancer
Winner,* about her healing of melanoma when she had only
Gerson's book to guide her. What kept me plodding through
the religious effusions—she's a member of the Moral
Majority—was the strong indication of chemical toxicity, of
which she seemed unaware. This hint of a link between
cancer and chemicals—by no means the first—suggested to
me that cancer might be a symptom as much as a disease.

Although it was still early days, the regime was proving
less onerous than I anticipated, but then I seem to need a
tight framework in which to achieve anything at all. Perhaps
it was harder for those with stronger addictions to relinquish,
such as alcohol, tobacco, or drugs. Mine were the childish
cravings for chocolate and carbohydrates, but no less
tenacious for that. Alas, the road to health is paved with
renunciation.

During Charlotte's visit on the 29th, I told her about my
swollen foot and the suture that had been left in one toe.

"That reminds me of a patient whose nose began to swell
at the start of the therapy," she said. "Shortly thereafter, a
suture appeared in one nostril. When I asked if she'd had a
nose operation, it turned out that she'd had a rhinoplasty

thirty years earlier. She recalled that, two weeks after the operation, a small piece of suture stuck out from inside her nostril. Instead of pulling it out she had cut it off, and, since it hadn't bothered her, she forgot about it. Because the therapy helps the body expel any hostile substance, the tissue surrounding the remaining suture became inflamed and it made its way out of her body quite naturally.

"By the way," she added, "how many operations have you had—I mean with drugs and antibiotics?" When I told her five in one year, her hands flew to her face in mock horror. "Thank God they didn't give you chemo when you had cancer," she said, "because it destroys what is left of the immune system, which makes it much harder for the therapy to work."

I remembered a question I meant to ask, although I thought I knew the answer.

"I read in the primer, Charlotte, that patients are warned to take care of any dental work prior to embarking on the therapy. Why is that?"

"It's because the detoxifying body is too sensitive to tolerate anesthetic."

I told her of my near-death experience in Dallas, adding, "I understand the ECU has since been closed and Dr. Rae now has a sauna program instead."

"Well, saunas can sweat out some of the toxins," she said, "though not all can be eliminated through the skin."

"I wonder why I felt so well after the four-day fast, only to have my symptoms return when I started eating single-food meals?"

"That's because your body was still full of poisons. Fasting gives temporary relief to an overloaded system, but it should not be applied in chronic disease because deficiencies are always present. My father opposed fasting as a detoxification procedure, since it doesn't restore the urgently needed minerals and vitamins to the organs. He didn't like spring water either—not only because much of it contains salt, but because the consistent purity of the spring cannot be guaranteed. There is no way to protect a spring from pollution."

On this subject Gerson was not only ahead of his time, he was wiser than he knew. At the 1984 convention of the American Dowsers Society in Vermont, a professional water diviner told us he had to go much deeper now than before to find potable water, because the underground aquifers are being contaminated by agricultural chemicals.[20]

More worrying than the poisoning of our food is the pollution of the world's water resources, for without pure water life on earth cannot be sustained.

As long ago as 1939, the French writer and aviator, Antoine de St. Exupery, wrote, in *Wind, Sand and Stars (Terre des Hommes)*:

> ... the human body cannot go three days
> without water. I should never have believed
> that man was so truly the prisoner of the
> springs and freshets. ... We believe that man
> is free. We never see the cord that binds him
> to wells and fountains, that umbilical cord by
> which he is tied to the womb of the world. Let
> man take but one step too many ... and the
> cord snaps.

That cord has been tightening for many years, yet only now have we begun to realize how soon it could snap.

I asked Charlotte if she was familiar with the hospice movement in England that was doing such wonderful work

---

[20] In 1985, there were over 60,000 contaminants in our wells. Alcalor and lindane had been found in 13,000. More than 45 million pounds of atrazine were sprayed onto fields each year. It seeped into streams that flow into the Missouri River, and ran into the groundwater from the streams. Three million people drank this water filled with higher concentrations of atrazine than the government standard, which is always too high and ignores the effect when two or more chemicals are ingested together.

for the terminally ill. At the word "hospice," she stiffened slightly and her manner changed.

"Yes, I'm familiar with the hospice movement," she said, "but that doesn't interest me." Seeing my evident surprise, she added, "You know Elisabeth Kübler-Ross?"

"Of course." Kübler-Ross's work in helping the dying come to terms with death was legendary even in the 70's. It was at her lecture in London on *Death and Dying* that I learned of the hospice movement, which was pioneered in England by Dame Cicely Saunders.

"Now Kübler-Ross is a wonderful woman," said Charlotte, "a *caring* woman, who is breaking down the taboos about death." She paused. "But I would not let her set *foot* in this place!"

Her vehemence shocked me. How could *she,* of all people, be so uncaring?

"I don't understand, Charlotte, why wouldn't you?"

"Because I'm not interested in helping people to *die!*" she said, spitting out the word as if it were an ugly oath. "We're only interested here in helping people to *live!*"

The way she said *"live!"* was so triumphant, so life-affirming, it made me want to stand up and cheer. If Charlotte Gerson was a chip off the old block, what a Sequoia the block must have been!

Norman Frye's lecture that afternoon focused on Max Gerson's life, which had been one of high achievement plagued by tragic misfortune. Beata describes it so engagingly in her book that, with her permission, I am quoting part of it here:

> From my sketchy sources he came across as a strong, gentle, quiet man, absorbed in his work, absent-minded enough to wreck four bicycles in minor accidents and to fall down a coal chute. Above all he was modest, unpretentious and tenacious. Without exceptional staying power he might have packed up medi-

cine altogether or suffered a breakdown in his prime, for his whole life was punctuated by tragic reverses and disappointments. It was as if Fate had offered him marvelous opportunities with one hand, only to snatch them back with the other just before fruition. Yet even with such a cruel stop-go pattern Dr. Gerson had achieved unique results; what might he have done on a smoother track?

Two episodes of his career stood out as particularly bitter milestones. In 1932, when he was fifty-one, he was granted full facilities at a Berlin hospital to prove that his dietary treatment could cure even hopeless cases of tuberculosis. After long and painstaking efforts he was due to demonstrate his results before the Berlin Medical Association, in a presentation that, he knew, would make his therapy widely accepted and open the door to further pioneering work. But five weeks before the scheduled demonstration Hitler came to power and Dr. Gerson left Germany with his wife and three daughters. (Many of his relations who refused to follow his example perished in Nazi concentration camps.)

Another dazzling opportunity came—and went—in 1946 when Dr. Gerson, by then resettled and working in New York, was allowed to present five of his recovered cancer patients to a US Congressional committee, the first physician to be able to do so. What was at stake was a Senate Bill that, if passed, would have provided funds for research into his therapy. The presentation was an unqualified success, but the lobby supporting conventional cancer therapies defeated the bill by four votes. And that was that. The solitary immigrant doctor with his German-flavoured

English and remarkable results was once more left out in the cold, partly ignored, partly persecuted by various medical organizations, including the American Cancer Society, which listed his therapy under the heading of 'Frauds and Fables.' But he went on working, alone, amid increasing difficulties, and died at the age of seventy-eight, in 1959. As the final irony of his strange fate, the New York Academy of Science invited Dr. Gerson to become a member—two months after his death.

Only once did his life pattern seem to have worked in reverse when, instead of reducing a great chance to ashes, it turned a severe handicap into a tool of discovery. As a young man Dr. Gerson suffered from long, incapacitating bouts of migraine which his medical colleagues could not cure. So he began to experiment with various diets and soon found that a saltless regime of raw or freshly cooked vegetables and fruits, especially apples, banished his migraines. He recommended the same diet to his migraine-stricken patients, with excellent results. Soon one of those patients reported that his severe attacks of migraine had ceased—and his *Lupus vulgaris* (skin tuberculosis) was also healing. Since *Lupus* was considered incurable, Dr. Gerson could hardly believe the man's claim—or the evidence of his own eyes. But there could be no doubt. The *Lupus* lesions were healing. And he was forced to conclude that the diet was not so much healing a specific illness as restoring the body's own ability to heal itself—of migraine, *Lupus,* TB, or whatever was wrong with it. That was how his revolutionary work began, leading, in due course, to his startling success with terminal cancer cases.

When Gerson immigrated to America in 1936, he was 55 years old and spoke little English. To pass the New York State board examination, he went to school with first- and second-grade children to learn the language. He obtained his medical license in January, 1938.

After his presentation before Congress was defeated, the *Journal of the American Medical Association* (*JAMA*) reported, "Fortunately for the American people, this presentation received little, if any, newspaper publicity." In January 1949, the same journal stated, "There is no scientific evidence whatsoever to indicate that modifications in the dietary intake of food or other nutritional essentials are of any specific value in the control of cancer." Thirty years later, the AMA was still claiming, "There is no proof that diet is related to disease."

Efforts to destroy Gerson did not stop at his therapy alone. Twice, he became violently ill after being served coffee by a group of people he was led to believe were supporting him. Laboratory tests showed arsenic in a 24-hour sample of his urine. Some of his best case histories disappeared mysteriously from his files. Then, in 1956, someone stole his almost-completed book manuscript.

Gerson was 75 years old and faced with rewriting his entire life's work. *A Cancer Therapy: Results of Fifty Cases* was published in 1958. In the fall of that year, he realized that, at 77, and in failing health, he would never finish his next book, which would present 100 more recovered cancer cases. He died of pneumonia in March 1959. Even then, the medical establishment claimed he had died of cancer, ignoring his death certificate, which confirmed the cause.

How many life-saving cures were lost in the gas ovens of the Nazi extermination camps? What eminence might Gerson have achieved had he not been driven from his native land? Like so many pioneers, he was an eccentric genius—

unable, or unwilling to conform to the prevailing norm. Such men and women are too single-minded to care about image and too honest to cultivate charm. They can also be prickly challengers of the status quo. Scorned by their peers and denied funding during their lifetimes, after they die their discoveries are appropriated (without credit) and hailed as "new" by the sort of people who, when they were alive, would have dismissed them as quacks.

Not much has changed since Gerson's day. The obstacles he faced in 1946 confront the heretical visionary today. Medical McCarthyism still flourishes, with greed and power suppressing cures that threaten the enormous profits of the cancer industry—a cartel that continues to tell thousands of sufferers, "There is no cure, but one is on the way."

Frye's lecture that day ended with a description of the latest craze of the 1980s: fire-walking.

"It encourages people to run barefoot over burning coals as a means of conquering their fear," he explained. "Once you've done that—conquered a different kind of fear—you have more courage with which to face your cancer."

Well, perhaps. But cancer didn't scare me in 1974. Compared to the kind of fear I had lived with these past six years, skipping barefoot over hot coals was a game for masochistic morons.

"I will show you fear in a handful of dust," wrote T.S. Eliot: in the chemical spray from a crop-duster's plane; in the toxic particulates that waft through the air, and in the mushroom cloud that may one day spread its nuclear death over us all.

CHAPTER TWENTY-THREE

Great spirits have always encountered
Violent opposition from mediocre minds.
—Albert Einstein

Two newcomers appeared at our dinner table on the 29th, a quiet young man who suffered from asthma and his guitar-playing companion, a Texas evangelist in his thirties.

"Hi, there!" said the latter, rising mid-meal to address the room. "My name's Jimmy Jackson—*Pastor* Jimmy Jackson—and this here is my friend, Roy, who's the patient. I understand it's someone's birthday today. Could y'all raise your hand, whoever you are? Oh, it's you over there. Well, c'mon, everyone, let's all sing 'Happy Birthday' to the birthday girl."

He seemed an odd companion for his reticent friend, who said scarcely a word during dinner. With his guitar, his soft baby face and brown hair combed in an upstanding quiff, Jimmy Jackson seemed more Elvis than evangelical.

"I'd like you to know," he added in his Texas twang, "that if I can be of help to any of you while I'm here, I'd be glad to oblige. Oh, and I'll be having a sing-along in the lounge after dinner, for any of you who'd care to join me."

"Shall we go to my room now, Nora?" I asked. My typewriter developed a glitch that afternoon, and being electronically thick, I issued a distress call during dinner. To my surprise, Nora said she was quite good at fixing things and offered to have a look at it. David, who had been quieter than usual that evening, said he would return to their room.

It took Nora only minutes to detect the portable's problem and put it to rights, while I looked on in bewildered admiration. We then sat on the bed for a while and had a quiet talk together.

"I'm so worried about David," Nora confided. "He's not doing at all well. I think his cancer is too advanced to be helped by anything now. If only we had known about this option before he was given so much chemo." She paused, and gazing somewhere in the middle distance, said, "We've been married for thirty-six years. It won't be easy . . . letting him go."

I reached for her hand, wondering why shared sorrow brings us so much closer than shared joy. It was hard at such moments not to rail at the injustice of fate, the nearness of death, and the remoteness of God. Hindered by the inadequacy of words, I had only banalities to offer her. As we were talking, I felt a queer illness steal over me. My thoughts grew muddled and I kept losing the thread.

"Are you all right?" asked Nora, noting my confusion.

"I think so—that is, I don't know. I'm feeling a bit odd."

"Perhaps you should lie down. Would you like me to call a nurse?"

"No, no, it will pass. Anyway, David needs you; Nora. He seemed to be having a hard time at dinner this evening. But thank you again . . . for everything . . . ."

After she left, I stretched out on the bed and interrogated my body. Was this a chemical flare-up? If so, it wasn't a very big one. I just felt sick and unconfident and alone.

A coffee break eased the discomfort and I returned to Jaquie Davison's book. Reading of the strong family support she had while doing the therapy—a sympathetic husband and a daughter who took a year off school to make the juices for her mother—I realized why the regime will never be widely used as it now stands, for to succeed three things are essential:

1. Sufficient funds to pay for the juicer, supplements and food.

2. Someone to make the juices and meals—a full-time, labor-intensive job.

3. Family support—or, failing that, the courage to go it alone.

Lacking any one of these, success is unlikely. It in no way diminishes Davison's achievement to say that without her strong support system at home, the outcome might have been very different.

On the 30th of August, the niacin flush made my bottom go all crimson, like the bum of those exotic monkeys in zoos who display themselves to sniggering schoolchildren. I still didn't know if I'd had a proper flare-up, apart from devastating fatigue on castor oil days.

"Don't you feel lonely down there in the annex?" Nora asked me the next day as we were finishing lunch. "You're missing a lot, you know, by not being in the upper building. Why don't you take our room when we leave day after tomorrow? It's larger than yours and much nicer. Then, too," she added, "you'd be closer to the nurses in case of an emergency." Seeing the wry smile this comment elicited, she said, "Well, suppose you had an emergency at night down there, all by yourself?"

"Oh, Nora, what could a nurse do for me, even if she spoke English? They deal with cancer here, not chemicals."

"But I don't like to think of you being so alone down there."

Just then, Jimmy Jackson rose to make an announcement.

"Good afternoon all. I'll be having a musical get-together after lunch, for any of you who'd care to join me."

"Very well, Nora," I said, "let's have a look at your room." As we were leaving the annex, I added, "Oh, by the way—I hope your room isn't near his."

"Oh, no," she assured me. "They're four doors away. Anyway, I was told he's been asked not to play the guitar in the evening, because the patients need rest and quiet."

"Well, that's a mercy," I said. But then, afraid of sounding judgmental, I added, "He's not a bad chap; it's just that I

153

lived for a month with a Baptist woman in Texas and a little fundamentalism goes a long way."

The upper level was indeed more spacious than the annex, with a broad tiled corridor and chairs that invited communal visiting. On reaching their room, I was brought up short by the sign on the door:

GOD IS LOVE

Noting my surprise Nora explained, "It was left there by a previous occupant. You can remove it, if you wish."

"I wouldn't dream of removing it," I said. "I used to see those words every Sunday in church. They were engraved on a plaque behind the lectern; they make me feel right at home."

In addition to being larger and nicer than my cubicle in the annex, their room had a water cooler inside and ample space for the desk. More compelling, however, was the thought of Nora and David's vibrations surrounding me when they were gone. It would mitigate to some extent the sadness I felt at their leaving.

The postprandial lecture that day was given by a German-born woman, Hildegard, who Charlotte described as "one of the sickest patients we've ever had." She visited the clinic once a week to inspire patients and instruct them on how to reorganize their kitchens after they return home.

Hildegard told us her cancer began with a tumor in her thymus the size of a grapefruit.

"When the doctors opened me up to remove it, they found that the tumor had invaded not only my thymus but my chest cavity as well. It had attached itself to my heart, the aorta, trachea, and sternum. Since my condition inoperable, they took a biopsy, closed me up, and gave me radiation—5,000 rads of cobalt to the thymus alone.

"After three weeks of this, I became violently ill, had severe burns on my esophagus and difficulty swallowing. The radiation caused my right lung to collapse and I developed pericarditis. My heart sac was full of pus, I had edema in my legs and throughout my body, and a liver scan taken in 1977 showed spots of cancer."

When Hildegard came to the clinic, the doctor told her that not even the Gerson Therapy could help her and advised her to go home. But she said, "No, I've come here to get well and I'm going to stay."

When she began the therapy in February 1979, she had hair loss, an enlarged liver, an immovable shoulder, a collapsed lung, and fluid in her lower lung and heart. Now, six and one-half years later, and in her fifties, Hildegarde was the picture of health.

"I teach, work, and walk five miles or more every day. I do all my own housework and am about to go on a sailing trip with my son. If *I* could make it," she told us confidently, "so can you."

Yes, I thought, but only if we have your courage and determination.

On September 1st, I woke with strange new aches and pains in different parts of my body. I had skipped the last coffee break the night before, because it was too hot and I was too tired. I had gone off food as well and was sorely tempted to cheat on the juices; but conscience kicked in and I forced them down. This therapy was no mañana affair.

After a sad good-bye to Nora and David in the morning, I began to pack for the move to their room. There were too many stairs to the upper level for me to carry my suitcase, typewriter and air purifier alone, so I rang the office for help. A girl appeared at the door and said a muchacho would come shortly to help with the cases.

While waiting for him to arrive I went to see Randy, whose room was two doors down from mine. He hadn't been to the dining room for two days and his absence caused concern at our table. I knocked gently and a young woman opened the door.

"Hello," she said, "I'm Randy's wife. My brother-in-law needed a break, so I came to take over. I'd invite you in, but he's not up to seeing anyone, I'm afraid. He's been in

155

constant pain, lying on his stomach for the past two days, because one buttock is terribly swollen. He's been coughing up blood and his bed linens can't be changed because he's too ill to be moved."

Seeing my eyes slide down to the small knife in her hand, she gave an apologetic little laugh.

"Oh, this," she said. "I've been cutting grapes into a bowl and applying them as a poultice to the inflamed places on his body. Well," she sighed, "when you're desperate, I guess you'll try anything."

Yes, I thought, as I walked back to my room, desperation brought all of us here, some to find healing while others— often, it seemed, the most worthy—to find the journey began too late. I recalled an axiom my father liked to recite when he caught me feeling sorry for myself:

> I wept because I had no shoes,
> Until I met a man who had no feet.

When an hour had passed with no sign of a muchacho, I went to the kitchen to see if they could find someone to help. Eventually, a man whose muchacho days were long past arrived. I followed him up the stairs with my typewriter and air purifier. He said he would bring the desk later, but I never saw him again. Moving day, Mexican style, was pretty much a do-it-yourself affair.

On September 2nd, Dr. Melendez brought me the results of my standard blood test. It was normal, but showed low thyroid and a weak immune system.

"We'll have to do another blood test to see if your lymphocytes have gone up," she said. "These are the white cells that fight infection and disease. They should be between 20 and 40, but yours are below 10. So you'll have to remain on the full therapy."

"Splendid," I said. "Precisely what I intended to do."

Meanwhile, the pastor's presence was beginning to cloy. Chatty and exuberant, unburdened by doubt or humility, he played his guitar, sang hymns and offered his spiritual counsel to one and to all. Some of us were giving him a wide berth. Returning to my room after the lecture that day, I caught a glimpse of J.J. on the first floor, surrounded by the girls from the kitchen, singing a song whose lyrics consisted solely of *Vaya con Dios,* ad infinitum.

The move to the upper building proved to be a mixed blessing, the gain in space offset by the thinness of the walls, through which I could hear every movement in the neighboring room, every footstep in the corridor, and every knock on someone else's door.

Two nights later, I was kept awake by the sound of muffled voices and laughter in the next room. I was reaching for my earplugs when the twang of a guitar brought me bolt upright in bed. *Oh, no, God,* I cried; *you couldn't do this to me! Who can he be visiting at this hour? It's nearly ten!* I shoved in my earplugs and buried my head in the pillow, muttering darkly, *Who will free me from this turbulent pastor?* Someone Up There must have been listening, for a few minutes later, J.J. packed it in.

I was drifting off to sleep when a trolley came clattering down the corridor and stopped outside my window. Two maintenance men had chosen this hour to replace a light bulb in the ceiling—a task that required much animated discussion and repositioning of the ladder on the tiled floor.

Yielding to the inevitable, I shoved the earplugs in further, wrapped the pillow around my head and wished fervently that I had never left the annex.

CHAPTER TWENTY-FOUR

*It is conceivable that man may have to set an
arbitrary limit to his domain—draw a line
where he ends and God begins.*
—E.B. White

I was leaving for breakfast the next morning, when I
noticed an odd sign hanging on my neighbor's doorknob—
the room J.J. was visiting the night before. It pictured a large
set of headphones encircling the words, TUNED IN TO
GOD! When I returned an hour later, the sign was reversed.
It now said, LISTEN! THERE'S GOOD NEWS IN JESUS!
The clinic was simply athrob with religious zeal.

Charlotte's postprandial talk that afternoon began by
addressing the subject of stress.
"Stress does not cause disease," she said, flatly. "If it did,
we would all be sick. It *can* be a precipitating factor if the
body is already not functioning well and is deficient and
toxic. Then, the addition of stress can be the straw that
breaks the camel's back. But in a normal, healthy body,
stress alone does not cause disease."
Returning to the subject of nutrition, she explained,
"Chronic disease has two basic factors: deficiency and
toxicity. Deficiency comes from our food, which is altered,
processed, manufactured, canned, frozen and so on. The vital
live substances are gone. Toxins are enzyme inhibitors; so is
sodium. Doctors in medical school aren't given courses in
biochemistry and that's where the healing occurs. If correct

nutrition can cure terminal cancers, imagine how few cancers there would be if we followed a healthy lifestyle from the start. Most of us are walking about in a state of half-health, believing ourselves to be well because we are not yet actually sick.

"And here I would like to say a word about soy. Soy is not a healthy food. It is a toxic by-product of the vegetable oil industry. Before soybeans reach your table, Hexane or other solvents have been applied to help separate the oil from the beans, leaving trace amounts of these toxins in the commercial product. This substance blocks the absorption of any and all nutrients you take in. It also causes cancer of the thyroid. All soybean products contain trace amounts of carcinogenic solvents. They also contain much fat, thus stimulating tumor growth."

Charlotte closed her lecture that day with a humorous story about a patient who had been on the therapy since her child was born.

"The patient's daughter was still young when she went to a friend's house for her first overnight stay. On returning home the next morning, the little girl said to her mother, 'You know, Mommy, they do the strangest things with coffee in her house—they *drink* it!'"

After the lecture, I returned to the upper building and was about to enter my room, when a voice said, "Hi there. I've got a surprise for you!" I turned to see Jimmy Jackson approaching. "You've got new neighbors," he beamed, producing a key and inserting it in the door with the Jesus sign. My heart sank.

"You mean . . . this is *your* room?" I stammered.

"That's right."

Dear Jesus, I thought, *this is not good news. Nora promised me!* I managed to smile and said, with as much grace as I could muster, "Well, I hope you won't be playing the guitar at night, Jimmy, because I turn in early and I'm a light sleeper."

"No problem," he said cheerfully. "If there's anything I can do for you, just let me know." He flashed a winning, if wasted smile and we entered our adjoining rooms.

True to his word, Jimmy did not play the guitar that night. He played it the next day—and sang—with his door open: *"Drop Kick Me, Jesus, through the Goal Posts of Life!"*

For several days I lived in peaceful coexistence with my neighbor. If I was dressing or recording the day's events in my diary the occasional riffs next door didn't bother me. But if I was trying to read, or work, or think, it turned my brain into porridge. I could ignore the voices and laughter, even the odd sonorous belch, but music—*my* kind of music, that is—was such a visceral part of my life I couldn't tune it out, much less ignore the sort I would have gone some distance to avoid.

On the morning of September 4th, I tried everything I could think of to muffle the sound: ear plugs, setting the air purifier on "high," cursing the wind, but even when muted, those lachrymose twangs made the effort to think like a slow tread through treacle. After reading the same paragraph in *Many Mansions* twice, without taking in a single word, my tolerance threshold finally was breached. There was nothing for it but to Take Steps.

I marched into the corridor, knocked on J.J.'s open door and entered. He was reclining on the bed in a red dressing gown, strumming idly on the guitar. Roy sat sprawled in the armchair, doing nothing in particular.

"Forgive me, Jimmy," I began, "I know I'm not as ill as most of the patients here, but I *am* desperately in need of peace and quiet. If you must play the guitar, would you mind playing it somewhere else or moving to another room? I think there's an empty one at the end of the corridor."

Jimmy set the guitar to one side, propped himself up on his forearm and studied me with a level gaze.

"I know there's an empty room at the end of the corridor," he said, "'cause that was our room before we moved here. But *you* can move, if you like," he added, a touch ungraciously, I felt.

"With the greatest respect, Jimmy, I'm a patient here and you're not. I'm simply asking you to show some consideration. By the way, may I ask *why* you changed your room?"

"We had to move 'cause there was no water in the shower and we got tired of waiting three days for it to get fixed."

"I see," I said. There was no answer to that, so after securing his promise of restraint I returned to my room, cursing Mexican plumbing, cursing the mañana culture, and cursing my intolerably low noise threshold.

Frye's lecture that afternoon focused on the emotional flare-ups we could expect in the months ahead.

"Anger, lethargy, discouragement, depression—these are all part of the body's vigorous efforts to detoxify itself," he warned. "They can begin at any time. Some start a few days into the therapy while others not for several weeks. But the first are usually the worst."

I thought of the ten-day fury Beata experienced during her stay at the clinic. In her book, she writes that it made her regret the loss of self-control that enabled her to deny and repress her anger—"lashing out verbally, with deadly precision, only when the provocation grew too strong." As an occasional, if unwitting, provocateur, I could attest to her deadly precision.

The anger flare-up, however, was one I was unlikely to have. Growing up with a father who was given to unpredictable rages, I learned early on to keep my own anger firmly battened down. My way of coping was to withdraw into a quiet place within and curl up with denial.

I was sitting next to Pearl, whose gum-chewing asides I tried to ignore, while on my right was a man in his seventies who I had seen walking in the corridor outside my room. A tall, gaunt figure with a pronounced stoop, he had to stop every few steps and breath heavily, as if to replenish his lungs.

161

"... And now," Frye was saying, addressing the environment, "most of the world's topsoil is gone, washed into the sea as a result of our mismanagement of earth's limited resources ...." He stopped suddenly, for an unpleasant odor had invaded the room.

"Jesus!" croaked Pearl, "what's that smell?" We glanced out the window and saw a man with a tank on his back spraying the lawn near the building. "Ye Gods!" shrieked Pearl, "it's pesticides!"

A strangled sound to my right made me turn.

"I've got to get out of here," gasped the old man, who was struggling for breath. "I have lung cancer . . . I can't take this."

"Neither can I," I said, feeling my own lungs begin to constrict, "let's go!" I took his arm and we headed toward the door, Frye's lecture forgotten in the ensuing consternation. Mounting the stairs as fast as his legs and lungs would allow, we reached his room, where he hooked himself up to the oxygen tank that stood in the corner. I waited until his breathing eased before returning to my room, for by then I, too, was in need of oxygen. There should have been a cylinder in the hall, but it had disappeared, so I rang for one.

When it finally arrived, the plastic mask smelled so strongly of polyvinyl chloride, that whatever benefit I might have obtained from the oxygen would have been vitiated by the outgassing chemical. (The masks in the ECU were ceramic and the hose made of Tygon—polyurethane tubing—which is odorless.)

By dinnertime, I had recovered enough to descend to the dining room, only to find that it, too, was filled with the same chemical odor. What madness has overtaken this place? I wondered. How could Charlotte *allow* such poisons to be sprayed near patients who were terminally ill?

"Do you know what that stuff was they sprayed here today?" said Randy, whose appearance at dinner that evening was a heart-lifting surprise. "It was Malathion. I recognized it 'cause we've used it on the farm."

"But Malathion is supposed to be safe," said Morris.

"Not for people with cancer it's not safe," said Randy. "They've been spraying the kitchen, too, so now all our good organic food is probably contaminated as well. Hell!" he exclaimed, throwing down his napkin in disgust. "This whole damned place is contaminated! I'm going to have my dinner sent to my room."

He stood up and, leaning heavily on his wife's arm, made his way to the door. I followed soon after, for my fingers were flaring and my breathing was becoming labored. *What on earth are we doing to the planet?* I wanted to shriek. *What, in God's name, are we doing to ourselves?*

Half a century ago, Rachel Carson warned us about Malathion:

> The alleged "safety" of Malathion rests on rather precarious ground, although—as often happens—this was not discovered until the chemical had been in use for several years. Malathion is "safe" only because the mammalian liver, an organ with extraordinary protective power, renders it relatively harmless. The detoxification is accomplished by one of the enzymes of the liver. If, however, something destroys this enzyme or interferes with its action, the person exposed to Malathion receives the full force of the poison.
>
> Unfortunately for all of us, opportunities for this sort of thing to happen are legion. A few years ago a team of Food and Drug Administration scientists discovered that when Malathion and certain other organic phosphates are administered simultaneously, a massive poisoning results—up to fifty times as severe as would be predicted on the basis of adding together the toxicities of the two. In other words, one-hundredth of the lethal dose

of each compound may be fatal when the two are combined.[21]

The Malathion exposure set me back a week in the therapy. Exhaustion, hypersensitivity, panicky feelings—all had returned. When I ran a comb through my hair, it flew away from my head as though I had stuck my finger in a live electrical socket or had seen a ghost. Dismayed at this setback, I looked up "pesticides" in Gerson's book and found the following paragraph:

> . . . Pesticide and herbicide spraying any-where near the home is devastating to the healthy body, much more to the debilitated healing body. Equally toxic is water pollution with fluorides, herbicides, pesticides, nitrates, silica and arsenic, etc. The patient cannot heal properly if the body continues to be contami-nated.

The next morning on my way to breakfast, I looked in on the old man to see how he was. I found him dressed, but sitting listlessly in his chair.

"I'm still having respiratory problems," he said, breath-ing heavily, "although my primary cancer is in the prostate. My back has been hurting me something terrible, too, but that's probably because of my job."

"Oh? What do you do?"

"I'm a carpet cleaner by profession, but for the last few months I've been laying carpets—been on my hands and knees a lot, you know, bending over."

I caught my breath. Not only had this gentle man been breathing chemicals all his life—for months he'd been inhaling their toxic vapors at close range![22]

---

[21] A recent study by Dartmouth University showed that, when you combine just one pesticide with one other pesticide, the toxicity increases by 150 to 1,600 times.

I thought back to the day wall-to-wall carpeting was installed in my flat and the devastating illness that felled me that same night. After I learned how chemicals outgas from new carpeting, I checked my diary for the date the carpet was laid and confirmed that collapse followed installation.

"Have you ever considered," I asked, carefully, "that your cancer might have been caused by the chemicals you've been working with and breathing in all your life?—the chemicals in carpeting, I mean."

"Why no," he said. "It's never occurred to me."

I gazed into his kind, trusting eyes and wanted to weep for his innocence. Would the day ever come when new carpets carry a government health warning:

THE CHEMICALS IN THESE CARPETS CAN BE
HAZARDOUS TO YOUR HEALTH!

When Charlotte came to my room the next day, I began to tell her about the Malathion, but she had already been briefed.

"That should *never* have happened," she said, angrily. "But you see, the Mexican government has a law that all public buildings and private institutions must be sprayed once a month."

"Once a month! But that's insane!"

"Of course it is. Which is why we've had an 'arrangement' to ensure that no spraying will be done inside our front gate. Something must have gone wrong yesterday. I'm terribly sorry. But I should explain that I'm not in control here. I don't own the clinic."

"You don't? I thought you did."

---

[22] There are almost 1,000 different chemicals in synthetic carpeting, apart from the styrene-butadiene latex backing and polyurethane foam underlay. Tests conducted in January 1993 by the Environmental Protection Agency showed that, when five mice were exposed to air blown over carpet samples, four mice died after suffering neurological disorders. EPA (1993).

"No, it's owned by the Mexican doctors who run it. Foreigners aren't allowed to have a clinic in Mexico, unless Mexicans own it. My position here is only an advisory one. I can suggest, but I cannot enforce."

Then that explained the shambolic attitude to hygiene that was so prevalent in the clinic, and so un-Germanic—such as the closet door I rarely saw closed during my three-week stay; a door that bore the sign:

FAVOR MANTENIR CERRADA LA PUERTA;
QUARTA SEPTICO!
(Please keep this door closed; septic area!)

We discussed the prevailing ignorance of government agencies about the systemic effects of chemicals and their threat to human health.[23]

"Almost everyone we see here who is suffering from motor neuron disease," said Charlotte, "has had insecticide poisoning. That's what insecticides are—neurotoxins."

"Motor neuron disease?"

"That's amyotrophic lateral sclerosis, or ALS," she explained, "better known as Lou Gehrig's disease. Sprays and inhaled toxins damage the brain and cause the motor neurons to malfunction. They also cause mental and emotional problems, including depression."

Her mention of ALS reminded me of the attractive woman I had seen at lunch that day. She could not have been more than fifty, but she was confined to a wheelchair and was being fed like a baby by a paid caregiver. Unable to talk or do anything for herself, her face was a study in frustration. If she needed something, the only way she could make the need known was to move her eyes in anguished entreaty, hoping the caregiver would be watching and able to interpret her meaning.

---

[23] There are 80,000 chemicals in production today, and more than 2,000 new chemicals are introduced each year. Only about 200 have been tested for safety. *Green America.*

I mentioned her plight to Charlotte, for I wondered at the woman's presence in the clinic.

"I doubt we can do much for her at this stage," she said. "Motor neuron disease is one of the worst things that can happen to a person. Melanoma? A *cinch* to cure by comparison. Give me a simple melanoma any day! What makes ALS so tragic is that the peripheral motor nerves and the muscles waste away, while the mind remains clear to the end. Body and brain stop communicating. You can't move, you can't speak, and eventually you can't even swallow. Each day you lose more control over your body—a body in which the mind remains trapped—until you finally choke to death. Compared with ALS, cancer is a snap, believe me!"

The realization that I might have had Lou Gehrig's disease instead of pan-sensitivity sent a shiver of fear through me, like the aftershock of a narrow escape. To be imprisoned in the body, unable to speak or read or do anything for myself—to be dependent on others for the rest of my life, all dignity gone and condemned to a slow, agonizing death . . . . Compared to that kind of torment, I, too, would prefer cancer—*any* affliction that would allow me at least to communicate, even if all I had to communicate was my despair.

CHAPTER TWENTY-FIVE

We have just enough religion to make us hate,
But not enough to make us love one another.
                                                        —Swift

By the 6th of September, the pastor's propinquity was becoming bothersome. Like a musical toothache his guitar throbbed in the corridor—joined, that morning, by a portable speaker through which he was favoring us with a tape of one of his sermons. Did the man never pray silently to his God? Is the Lord so deaf He hears us only when we shout? It used to be said in England that the landed gentry sent the fool of the family into the church. In America, the failed pop singer goes into evangelism.

When the sermon ended the strumming resumed. Driven to the end of my frail tether, I decided to go to J.J.—on bended knee, if necessary—and plead for some Christian mercy. Striding through the open door, I found him sitting on his bed in jeans and a striped T-shirt, practicing the passage that had me climbing the wall. Roy was in the bathroom, taking a shower.

"Jimmy," I began, "could you *please* play your guitar somewhere else? I love music, but when I need to work it shatters my concentration. I assure you that if you were the patient here and something I did was disturbing *you,* I would desist."

He gave me a long, penetrating look, the precise nature of which I could not determine. Then he placed his guitar on the floor, folded his hands in his lap and recited a passage from scripture—something about "whoever having this world's good and seeing his brother hath need, shutteth not up his bowels of compassion."

"Why, thank you, Jimmy," I said, disarmed. "I appreciate the generosity of spirit those words convey, I really do."

"That's okay," he drawled. "While you were talking the Lord spoke to me and said that I should do whatever I could to help a sister in need."

"Well, that's very good of you," I said, envying his hotline to God. Roy emerged from the bathroom, wearing a blue bathrobe and towel-drying his hair. "By the way, Jimmy," I added, "I've been meaning to ask you—how have you been able to take time away from your ministry to come here with Roy? After all, he doesn't appear to need a caregiver any more than I do."

"I came," said Jimmy, solemnly, "because Jesus told me I should come—to support a brother."

For one impious moment I wondered what had come over Jesus—sending Jimmy to try my soul, when he should be sending the halt and the sick. Suddenly, Jimmy asked, "Are you a practicing Christian?"

The question caught me off guard. Sensing we were on delicate ground, I chose my words carefully.

"I think I'm trying to be a practicing human being, but if you mean do I have a specific religion, the answer is 'no'—though I used to be a Christian Scientist."

"Oh, well, then," he said, dismissively, "you weren't really a Christian; Christian Science is just a cult."

Surprised at this description of my former faith, I asked Jimmy on what evidence he based his assessment. He reached for one of the leaflets on his nightstand and passed it to me. It was a church handout containing potted histories of four religions it claimed were doing the work of the devil, Christian Science being one. Intrigued, I read its version of the faith I had followed for thirty years.

"With respect, Jimmy," I said, returning it to him, "I'm afraid that whoever wrote this has got the wrong end of the stick. If they had done their homework, they would know that far from doing the work of the devil, Christian Science denies the very existence of that personage."

It was foolish to respond, of course—debates about religion are invariably futile. I would have enjoyed telling Jimmy about the poltergeist in our London flat and things that went bump in the night and invisible energy lines that respond to color and are found with a forked stick. If it was the devil and his works Jimmy was after, I could do him better than Christian Science. But he was trawling for souls and mine was clearly ripe for redemption.

"It's still just a cult," he said, ignoring my comment. "There's only one true faith and unless you become reconciled to God in the name of Jesus Christ and accept the Lord Jesus as your Savior . . . ."

"Forgive me, Jimmy," I interrupted, "but it *is* possible to have an abiding faith without having a specific religion."

"Without religion you can't be saved," he said, sternly. "Man is a sinner and needs to be saved. The Bible tells us so."

"Be that as it may," I replied, "it seems to me that, while there is much good in most religions, there is also so much bigotry and hate that, personally, I feel more comfortable with a one-to-one relationship with God. After all," I added committing the sin of pride by showing off all those years of Bible study, "'What does the Lord require of thee, but to do justly, and to love mercy, and to walk humbly with thy God?'"[24]

A look of infinite pity spread over Jimmy's face. Undaunted, I waffled on, resorting to the familiar metaphor of the mountain we're all climbing, though taking different paths, and that as long as we meet at the top . . . . But I could see from his face that my little homily was in no way getting me off the hook.

"Well," I concluded, a touch cravenly, "at least I'm not an atheist or an agnostic."

---

[24] Micah 6:8.

"In that case," he said, "I will pray for you. I will pray that you return to Jesus."

"Thank you, Jimmy," I said. "I'm not sure I've ever left him, but I can use all the prayers you've got."

On this note of conciliation, if not agreement, we ended our discussion and I returned to my room—Roy having remained mute the while.

Later, while trying to analyze what it was I found so irksome about the fundamentalists, I decided it was their awful sanctimony and relentless proselytizing. The trouble with born-again Christians is that they're even more tiresome the second time around.

There is something pitiless and hard in the belief that God speaks only to one group of people, while condemning the rest to eternal perdition. Wouldn't a truly loving Father want *all* His children to be saved? If there really were but one true faith, surely the millions who have been seeking it for millennia would have reached some consensus by now, instead of blowing each other to bits in sectarian wars.

At lunch the next day, Charlotte shared with us some of the problems the institute was facing at the time.

"The biggest problem is finding doctors to train in the Gerson method, since it's illegal in the U.S. for them to treat cancer with nutrition. Even those who've been cured by the therapy could lose their license if they recommend it to their patients."[25]

With a weariness that reflected the years of fighting to preserve her father's legacy, Charlotte added, "Little has changed since my father's day, when every article he submitted to *JAMA* was rejected for fear of losing its pharmaceutical advertisers. How could the journal give space to a doctor who cured cancer without drugs? What would become of the billion-dollar cancer research industry?" she

---

[25] There are now a number of Gerson practitioners in countries outside the U.S. For current information concerning licensed practitioners, see the Gerson website at www.gerson.org.

asked, pointedly. "It would be put out of business, that's what, its business being research more than finding a cure."

Indeed, Finding a Cure for Cancer is similar to The Second Coming: We've been told it will happen, we keep waiting for it to happen, but if it appears in a form different from the one we've been led to expect, we reject it.

And crucify it.

It seemed ironic that we have more freedom of religion in America than we do freedom of medical choice. The law protects a parent's right to withhold medical help from a child on religious grounds, even if it endangers the child's life, but a doctor who cures cancer by non-toxic means is left to the dubious mercies of a medical theocracy.

One of the signers of the Declaration of Independence, Benjamin Rush, MD, wrote, with far-seeing wisdom:

> Unless we put medical freedom into the Constitution, the time will come when medicine will organize into an undercover dictatorship. To restrict the art of healing to one class of man and deny privileges to others will constitute the Bastille of medical science. All such laws are un-American and despotic. . . . The Constitution of this Republic should make special provisions for Medical Freedom as well as Religious Freedom.

Hal was absent from the dining room that day, so after lunch I stopped by his room to see how he was getting on. To my surprise, I found him preparing to go home.

"But how will you manage the long plane journey, Hal?" I asked, wondering how he would survive the drive to the airport. "Won't you have two long flights with a stopover in between?"

"Yes, but I have to go. I've run out of money and besides, I don't think the therapy is helping me. I just want to go home and be with my family."

172

I longed to say, "Get thee to hospice," but didn't know if Australia had a hospice movement. Instead, hoping to give him a chuckle, I told him about my talk with J.J. the day before and the discovery that what I thought was my former faith was actually a cult.

Far from being amused, Hal took up where Jimmy left off and I found myself being hectored by a Seventh Day Adventist. Seizing his Bible, he proceeded to cite chapter and verse in support of Adventist belief. As far as I could make out, it is based on "the seven Cs," Christ being the first, the cross the second—and I've forgotten the rest.

"We go to church on Saturday instead of Sunday," Hal explained, "Saturday being the seventh day of the calendar, which is where our name comes from. And we believe The Second Coming is imminent. When you die," he added, with the rising fervor of a televangelist, "if you're a Christian, you'll be at peace when you join Christ in His heavenly mansion for a thousand years. The Christian dead will be the first to rise. All others will stay in the ground during the thousand years while Satan roams the earth with his evil angels, trying to convert those who remain to his evil power.

"None of your reincarnation rubbish!" he concluded scornfully, referring to a remark I let fall during an earlier visit.

Apparently, a thousand years in the heavenly mansion were preferable to an afterlife in which the mistakes made in this one might be redeemed. I couldn't help wondering what happened to the Christian dead when the thousand years were up. Were they turfed out of the mansion or could the lease be renewed? Prudence kept me from asking, for there was no warmth in Hal's philippic, no hint of humor or scintilla of doubt. And as Frances Wickes wrote, "Without the saving grace of doubt, man never arrives at the faith which is his own."[26]

By the time I said good-bye to Hal, I was so God-smacked I felt the whole world could do with a radical

---

[26] *The Inner World of Choice.*

theodectomy. It was a long time since I'd encountered so much rigidity of belief—"belief" in the sense of clinging passionately to something, whether the thing clung to is right or wrong. A bit of therapeutic blasphemy would be no bad thing, I felt. God can take it, even if some of His children can't.

But then, maybe Hal was having a flare-up.

Walking back to my room, I thought of the Buddhist story about God and Satan, who were walking together one day, when they saw a man ahead of them bend down and pick something up that glowed brightly in his hand. On seeing this, Satan gave a cry of delight.

Puzzled, God asked him what pleased him so?"

"That man has just found a piece of the truth," said Satan.

"But why should that make you happy?" asked God.

"Because," grinned Satan, "now, he's going to *organize* it!"

The more fervently the agents of God tried to hector me into holiness, the more grateful I was for the Founding Fathers—who, when framing the Constitution, took care to insure not only our freedom *of* religion, but our freedom *from* religion as well.

As E.B. White observed:

> Democracy is itself a religious faith, for some it comes close to being the only formal religion they have. And so when I see the first faint shadow of orthodoxy sweep across the sky, feel the first cold whiff of its blinding fog steal in from the sea, I tremble all over, as though I had just seen an eagle go by, carrying a baby.

CHAPTER TWENTY-SIX

Do I believe in God? Let's say
we have a working relationship.
—Noel Coward

On September 7th, I ran out of batteries for my tape recorder. Informed they could be found at *La Bottica,* one of the small shops across the street from the clinic, I set out on the short walk, eager to discover what amenities lay beyond our oasis.

Dodging the exhaust fumes of a passing car, I reached the other side of the road, where the shops stood like a hyphen between a PEMEX petrol station-cum-garage at one end and an old warehouse at the other. Large faded letters on the sloping roof of the warehouse read, *LAMINA DE ASBESTOS.*

I bought the new batteries at the liquor store—Duracell look-alikes that went dead after three days—and poked my nose into the adjoining shops to see what else was on offer. There was a store that sold cheap clothing and an all-purpose store where one could buy, among other things, the sort of food that must have given Dr. Gerson heartburn in his grave.

Yards away, a vendor was hawking tacos and chunks of gray meat that were bubbling in a vat of stomach-turning oil. It seemed hugely ironic that a cancer-curing therapy based on pure food and water had to find refuge in a country that ignored every principle on which it is based.

Between the last shop and the warehouse was a tall concrete wall with an arched opening that proved too tempting to resist. I stepped through it and found, stacked against either side of the wall, large sheets of asbestos, their flaking corners accessible to the fingers of any inquisitive child. What a reckless country this is! I thought—storing crumbling asbestos mere yards from where food and drink are being consumed. How many fibers had floated over the road to La Gloria? I wondered. How many patients, arriving with terminal cancer, went home with a little more asbestos in their lungs? At least Malathion warned you with its odor.

In his 1989 book, *High-Tech Holocaust*, James Bellini observed:

> In North America the old, developed world rubs shoulders with the newly industrialized; the first generation of acid polluters co-exists alongside one of the newest entrants to the league of contaminators. And it is the rise of younger economies such as Mexico, with their passion for development and lower regard for regulatory controls, that threatens to turn an already unacceptable level of world-wide acidity—the accumulated dross of a century of profligate old world frenzy—into a truly global eco-disaster.

I returned to La Gloria to find its own depredations continuing apace. On the way to my room, I passed a languorous worker stripping paint from the iron banister with a chemical that smelled like creosote. He was still at it when I went down to dinner, holding my nose as I rushed past him to avoid the fumes.

Worse was to come.

The floor of the administration building was awash with an odiferous foam, its fumes having made their way into the adjoining dining room. Halfway through dinner, I felt my worst symptoms returning. The real miracle of this place, I decided, was not that it cured cancer, but that it cured it in spite of chemical negligence on a monumental scale.

On the 8th of September, I was recording the day's events in my diary when a commotion in the corridor drew me away from my desk. I opened the door to see patients arranging chairs against the opposite wall, while a lanky, grey-haired gringo in his fifties positioned a group of Mexican children for some kind of performance.

"That's Dr. Long," explained a patient who had been at the clinic for several weeks. "He's an American. He teaches music at a religious mission in San Diego and comes to Mexico one day a week to give music lessons to the children. Once a month he brings them here to sing for us."

Delighted that my stay coincided with this event, I took a chair and was soon transported by the children's sweet, piping voices singing a cappella their native songs. Bright, upraised eyes followed their leader's hands as he varied the tempi with a restraining palm here, an encouraging sweep of the arms there, or a finger pressed to his lips for a final pianissimo.

At one point, the sudden thrum of a guitar made me twist around in my chair. There, framed in the doorway of his room, stood Jimmy—guitar strap slung over his shoulder, head bobbing in time with the music, while contributing a few superfluous riffs of his own. He was clad in his scarlet dressing gown, Elvis hair-do swept into a wavy tuft that fell over his forehead, and resembled nothing so much as a cocky cardinal—of both species.

At the concert's end Dr. Long and the children were acknowledging our applause, when Jimmy stepped forward to make a little speech of thanks on behalf of us all— bestowing upon the older man and his charges a blessing that would not have disgraced the Pope.

Two nights later, I lay awake in bed listening to the sounds in the next room—of drawers being opened and closed, objects being dragged across the floor and suitcases being snapped open and shut. My neighbors, I learned, would be decamping in the morning.

"Adios, Jimmy," I murmured, sliding happily under the covers. *"Vaya con Dios."*

Like everything else at La Gloria, the telephone system was capricious. With my stay at the clinic nearing its end, I had been trying to reach my daughter, Amy, at her home in Long Beach. She was to meet me at the San Diego airport on the 17th and drive me to Los Angeles for my flight back to London. I finally got through to her on the 16th, to let her know that a car would be taking me over the border early in the morning and the approximate time of our arrival.

That afternoon, Dr. Melendez came to my room to discuss the food I would be taking on the flight home the next day. Seeing me in bed, exhausted, she said, "Don't worry that you are tired. The exhaustion is a sign of the healing process as the toxins begin to enter your blood-stream."

"My only worry is that I might have a flare-up on the plane," I replied.

"Some flare-ups don't start until the fourth or fifth week," she said, in a kind but fruitless attempt to reassure me.

"But how will I know, when I'm having a flare-up in London, if it's a sign that I'm getting better or a sign that I'm getting worse?"

"You will know," she said, enigmatically. "Your body will tell you. Now, for the journey home you will have a thermos of soup, one of tea, one carrot juice, and two baked potatoes." It wasn't food that concerned me, it was having a migraine headache when I couldn't detoxify for fifteen hours or more. "The car will be here at 7:00 in the morning," Dr. Melendez concluded. "You will let me know of your progress when you return home, yes?"

"Oh, if only I could take you with me," I said, flinging my arms around her and feeling less confident than ever about the months ahead.

"I've just learned that Jaquie Davison has dyed her dark hair blonde again," said Charlotte that afternoon, during our final visit together, "even though she knows how dangerous hair dye is for those who've had cancer."

Foolish Jaquie, I thought, after all she went through to detoxify her "beautiful body." So much for "keeping our temple clean." It did make me wonder, though, about some of the people God saves, as against so many of those He lets die.

To Charlotte, I merely said, "It seems she had the experience but missed the meaning."

"She's crazy," shrugged Charlotte.

As I would be leaving at seven the next morning, I said my long good-byes after dinner to the few remaining patients with whom I had spent some time. Hal had returned to Australia—safely, I hoped—and Pearl had taken her husband home to Ohio. Morris would be staying on, of course, but Tina's future was uncertain. Indeed, some months after my return to London, I learned that she had died. As for Randy, my inner soothsayer could only weep for him and his family.

I had been feeling off-color all afternoon; not ill, exactly, but unaccountably anxious and on edge. While packing that evening, a cloud of depression descended upon me like a shroud. I couldn't think why. I wasn't sad about leaving; on the contrary, I couldn't wait to get home. I *was* apprehensive about the flight, but I had packed emergency needs in a carry-on, chiefly for the sense of security it gave me. Why, then, this mounting anxiety, this nameless pressure bearing down on my spirit?

By half-past ten, my heart was racing and I felt a funny vibration in my feet; it was as though a small battery was imbedded in the ball of each foot. The symptoms were similar to those I experienced when sleeping over a polluted stream or in a fractured energy line, only stronger. How could this be? I dowsed the room before leaving the annex and it dowsed clear.

The return of a sensitivity I had almost forgotten for three weeks alarmed me. I took out my Y-rod and explored the room again. It still dowsed quiet. Mistrusting the response, I picked up the color wheel to see if I could identify the source. Instantly! the rod went berserk—twisting and flipping over in my hands, as if reacting to every color in the wheel. The whole environment was a kaleidoscope of fractured energy lines. What on earth was causing this aberration? These energies weren't here before or I would have felt them.

A sudden panic gripped me as I realized that even here my condition was beyond help or understanding. With mounting anxiety I prayed, *Please, God, spare me this trial on the flight home!*

The night ahead loomed as dread-filled as all those nights I thought I had left behind in London. As midnight approached, my body went into overdrive; my feet throbbed, my fingers pulsed and my heart thumped wildly in its cage. I tried the oxygen tank. It was still in my room, though it shouldn't have been. It made no difference. My last coffee break was at ten. I took another. I drank some chamomile tea. I lay down, exhausted and longing for sleep, but my heart thumped so heavily I had to get up. Only by constantly moving could I prevent these energies, whatever they were, from boring through me like laser beams.

By midnight, my teeth were on edge and my scalp felt as though it was crawling with maggots. Needing to do something—anything—to distract my mind, I washed my hair. At half-past one I took a final coffee break, but it was no use; whatever this was, the therapy couldn't handle it.

I must have dropped off around 2:00 a.m., for when I woke at 5:00, I realized I had been asleep for three hours. I got up to go to the bathroom and glanced in the mirror—only to stare in disbelief at my reflection. My hair, which had been limp since the Malathion exposure, was standing in waves all over my head, just as it did in its crowning glory days. If this is a sign from God, I thought, it is one I will cling to in the months ahead.

Amy was waiting for me as my car pulled up at the airport. Even before her features came into focus, the sight of those ginger curls and faded jeans brought a lift to my heart. We hugged and kissed, and with her strong young arms around me, I felt reconnected to the world after my sojourn in the land of carrot juice and cancer.

We set off for Los Angeles, my born-again hair retaining its curl, so that I no longer needed the head scarf I resorted to before when in public. And now that my body was in motion again, those scary symptoms of the night before began to recede. By the time we reached LAX they were almost gone.

Sitting in the departure lounge with my daughter, chatting about her friends, her career in design and all the happy, trivial things that had nothing to do with the body and its ills, I began to feel like a normal person again. I had almost forgotten how hostile the outside world could be—until the smoke-filled air began to snake into my sinuses and I felt a headache coming on.

Amy had to leave before my flight was called. As we embraced good-bye, a great loneliness welled up inside. When would I see either of my daughters again—or my aging father? Would I be well enough next year to make my annual visit home?

After she left, my headache grew worse. It was as though a steel clamp was being tightened around my skull. My last coffee break had been eight hours ago and my body was on a four-hour schedule. If the pain is this bad now, I thought, what will it be like on the plane?

Desperate times call for desperate measures. A quick reconnaissance of the restroom confirmed a large stall for the disabled. I grabbed my carry-on, fetched some coffee from the dispenser in the lounge, topped it up with tap water from the sink in the Ladies' and locked myself in the loo. So what if the coffee wasn't organic or the water distilled.

The procedure was underway when someone entered the room. I lay very still, praying she wasn't disabled. Instead of using the facilities, however, she just stood there—doing what? I wondered. Putting on a full make-up from the sound of things. I heard the snap of a purse opening and the click of objects being placed on the counter, followed by long, agonizing stretches of silence in between. *Oh, go, please go!"* I prayed. *"What's taking you so long?*

At length, I heard her gathering her things together and the sound of the door opening, followed by the slow, sucking noise as it closed on her retreating footsteps. With a sigh of relief, I completed the operation and returned to the lounge. Even before my flight was called, the headache lifted.

We had been airborne for less than an hour when my hair collapsed again, its brief resurrection no match for the cabin's recycled air. With a heavy heart, I reached for the hated head scarf. I should have known the miracle was too good to last.

An hour later, the headache returned—this time with such a bone-crushing vengeance I wanted to hurl myself out of the plane. There was no way I could endure ten more hours of this agony or even ten more minutes. I staggered up the aisle and found a flight attendant in the galley. After describing my predicament, I asked,

"So is there by chance another loo on the plane a bit larger than the one in business class?" If the attendant thought me odd or my needs peculiar, she didn't let on.

"The one on the upper deck is slightly bigger," she said, pouring some coffee into a mug and handing it to me, "though not by much, I'm afraid."

I thanked her and with the mug in one hand, my carry-on in the other, I climbed the stairs to the deck above. The film had started, so with luck I would not be disturbed. I spread my trousers on the floor, adopted a tight fetal position—and, by the grace of God and Gerson, achieved the impossible. Within minutes of returning to my seat the headache was gone, this time for good, and I spent the rest of the flight in relative comfort.

Albert Schweitzer was right: Max Gerson *was* a medical genius. He was also, on this particular occasion, my savior in absentia.

Three weeks later, after the therapy was ticking over in London, I wrote to Charlotte:

"Am I the first Gerson person to negotiate a coffee break at 35,000 feet over the Atlantic?"

Her reply cut me down to size.

"Sorry," she wrote back, "another patient has beaten you to it."

Ah, well, the suffering I was spared that day meant far more than any entry in a Gerson Book of Records. Recalling all the high-flying headaches I endured in the past, I could only bless the doctor who saved me from what would have been the most agonizing journey of my life.

Dr. Gerson could hardly have imagined the lengths to which his therapy would be taken by a few patients who found themselves in extremis. Yet, such radical improvisation was no more than an extension of what he preached in his book—what Charlotte and Frye had stressed at La Gloria: namely, the importance of keeping the body detoxified— and, above all—the *vital* importance of taking responsibility for our own health.

CHAPTER TWENTY-SEVEN

The soil is our external metabolism. It is
not really far removed from our bodies.
—Max Gerson

My first week home was hectic, trying to maintain the rhythm of juices, meals, and enemas, while teaching the mechanics of the therapy to Isilda, the Portuguese helper I had engaged.

Short, squat, and tempestuous, Isilda tackled the kitchen chores with a vigor that made up in zest for what it lacked in equanimity. Her take-charge efficiency was a godsend, for it freed me to work on the book I was writing about my experience as an adopted child as well as adoptive parent. Eager to please, and immensely caring, Isilda was the proverbial treasure. That is, at first. Unfortunately, I hadn't foreseen the hazards of adding to my quiet way of life the live-in presence of a forty-five-year-old firebrand.

Deaf to noise and a stranger to silence, she banged doors, ran the vacuum cleaner under my feet while I worked, and flung cutlery into the kitchen drawer with such a clatter it was a job holding my thoughts together. Suspicious of all things mechanical, she took an instant dislike to the Norwalk juicing machine—a costly piece of equipment, irreplaceable in England, which I imported at great expense from the U.S. Dismissing the instruction book with a shrug, she jammed vegetables into the grinder with such ferocity that bits and pieces wound up all over the ceiling and cupboard doors.

"It really is quite simple to keep this from happening, Isilda," I said, showing her for the nth time how to keep the housing covered during the grinding process. But Isilda and simplicity were not on speaking terms.

"I do how you say," she replied irritably, "but the ve-ge-tables—they no like to stay in!"

It says much for the Norwalk's construction that it withstood twelve months of Isilda's abuse while churning out the enzyme-rich juices on which the therapy—and my hoped-for recovery—relied. I did sympathize, however, with her complaints about having to make ten juices a day (it should have been thirteen, but she had been warned).

Arriving at my desk with a glass of carrot juice, she would set it down as though it was hemlock, cross her hands over her apron and say, "I tell you this, my dear—all this juices is no good for your kidneys!" She was equally vocal in her disapproval of the salt-free, meat-free, organic meals she had to prepare.

"How you eat this food?" she demanded. "Is no taste! When I eat, make me sick!"

She was, of course, free to make for herself whatever her Portuguese palate preferred, but it did not take long to twig that Isilda was one of life's grumblers. At first her tetchiness amused me, for it was accompanied by a manifest eagerness to help me get well—as long as her help could be given in a way that *she* could understand.

"Tell me how I can *help* you!" she would cry over my prostrate form when I was in mid-flare-up and too ill, almost, to speak. Isilda could not understand that all I needed from her—all I wanted from her—was a steady flow of juices and support for what I was doing, whether she approved of it or not.

Convinced the therapy was making me worse, she would stand by my bed, arms akimbo on her sturdy hips, and say, "This thing you do—I no understand. I see you are in pain. You say, 'That is good.' When *I* have pain that is *not* good. It tell me something wrong. When you are sick, you say,

'That is good.' When you are *more* sick, 'That is better?' Is crazy therapy!"

"Yes, well, could we discuss it some other time, Isilda? Just give me until January and we'll see who's winning, the therapy or the pain."

At this, she would shrug and march out of the room. It was *my* loss if I refused her good advice and continued on this lunatic course.

While sifting through the mail that arrived during my absence, I came upon a flier that invited me, in exuberant type, to SKIP OVER HOT COALS TO CONQUER YOUR FEAR!—the same exercise Frye recommended at the clinic. Addressed, presumably, to the pain-deprived, it promised the discovery of courage through risking a slight burn on the soles of one's feet:

> This course enables people to transcend fear, to discover latent powers, do the seemingly impossible and use these skills in other areas of life.

I tossed it into the wastebasket. Been there, doing that now.

The 19th of September brought news of a huge earthquake in Mexico City that measured 8.1 on the Richter scale. As I read of the widespread damage and loss of life, I was ashamed of the relief I felt that the clinic was far enough away to have escaped the devastation.

The first unmistakable flare-ups began. A broken toe on my right foot started to swell. Painful calluses, similar to those that crippled me before, reappeared on the balls of my feet and an odd rash broke out on the tips of my fingers, causing the skin to peel away in ever-widening circles. Shooting pains in my scalp, stiffness in my neck and arrhythmic heartbeats were joined by a return of the sick-all-over-feeling and those scary tides in the head. Now, however, I understood—or rather, took it on faith—that they were proofs the detoxification process was underway. There were times when faith in Gerson had to be stronger even than faith in God.

When my fingers went numb one day, save for a faint tingling at the tips, I grew alarmed, for I heard this was a precursor of multiple sclerosis. During one such episode, I turned to the chapter on insecticides in Gerson's book and read:

> Areas of skin become exquisitely hyper-sensitive ... or irregular numbness, tingling sensations, itching or crawling sensations, or a feeling of localized heat may take place.

Further on, referring to experiments with insecticides conducted by the FDA as far back as the 1940s, he wrote:

> ... F.D.A. scientists have also shown that it is possible to store many times the amount in the body-fat that would be acutely fatal intra-venously in a single dose ... Cumulative in-toxication from extremely small amounts in food can thus be as dangerous as direct expo-sure to much larger amounts.

It was to hasten the exit of these cumulative toxins from the bloodstream that Gerson added coffee enemas to his regime. "Patients have to know," he wrote, "that the coffee enemas are not given for the function of the intestines but for the stimulation of the liver."

In 1985 organic vegetables in London were imported, expensive and in short supply. The only sources available to the few Gerson patients were a Whole Foods store on Baker Street and a supplier in Covent Garden—an amiable bandit, Ken, who shamelessly exploited our dependence on him for organic produce. Occasionally, he would slip a non-organic item into my order, on the reasonable assumption that I wouldn't notice the difference. My body did, however, and

187

alerted me to the imposter soon after its consumption. Eventually, I found an honest greengrocer in Chelsea—an Indian, whose prices were fair and whose organic vegetables, though limited, were displayed in their original cartons from Germany, curiously marked *Biologique* in French.

Four weeks into the therapy, on the afternoon of September 25th, my hair went limp, my fingers began to throb and my heart speeded up, skipping about erratically in my chest. Wondering what could be causing this relapse, I recalled that the day before, we ran out of organic carrots. To tide us over until Ken's delivery on the 26th, I bought five pounds of commercial carrots at the supermarket.

Acting on a hunch, I went to the kitchen where Isilda was preparing dinner.

"Isilda, when did you start using the new carrots?"

"This afternoon, last two juices. Why?"

"No reason, I just wondered." Best not to invite a sermon.

I had been reading *Silent Spring* again and came upon the following paragraph in my well-thumbed copy:

> Carrots absorb more insecticide than any other crop studied; if the chemical used happens to be lindane, carrots actually accumulate higher concentrations than are present in the soil.

Had Rachel Carson not died so tragically young, she might have included the more recent discovery that when commercial carrots are juiced, the pesticides become more concentrated in the juice. This may be the case when juicing all nonorganic vegetables and fruits.

Meanwhile, Isilda's care-giving, which at first was such a comfort, was beginning to feel more like a cross. Sometimes, when having a flare-up, I had to conceal from her how ill I really felt, if I wanted to avoid yet another exhortation to abandon the therapy. Finding me in mid-enema on the bathroom floor, she would plant herself in the doorway, all bossy briskness, and say, "I tell you, my dear—all this enemas is no good for your behind!" Or, "I tell you, my dear—this therapy you do—it make you crackers!"

Her disapproval notwithstanding, Isilda kept the juices coming and now that the regime was in full swing, I was surprised at how easily I adapted to its restraints. Averse to commitment and bored with routine, I embraced both as the price I had to pay for a restored immune system. My only fear was of having a flare-up the therapy couldn't handle, like the one that last night at the clinic; for if Gerson should fail, what then? To whom could I turn in a crisis? I had exhausted clinical ecology and my GP would just give me pills.

Only once did I weaken and break the rules. At the health food store one day, I lusted after a carob-coated rice cake. So I bought two and scoffed them both on the spot. Well, rice was safe, wasn't it? And carob better than chocolate?

Instantly, my hands turned red and my throat seized up. *Me, the unteachable self-punisher!* I moaned. Why did I think I could pull something over on my body? It was so much cleverer than I, and so vengeful. Stricken with shame, I fancied I could hear Dr. Gerson scolding me from his perch in the Pantheon:

"Well, if you won't stick to the rules, you deserve everything recidivism can throw at you."

Forgive me, Max. It won't happen again, I promise!

Locked as I was into my salt-free, sugar-free, fat-free, dairy-free diet, all the gustatory pleasures of the past were now a receding memory. Thanks to the therapy, however, I was able to stay in the flat at night, even though the energies that had driven me from it before were still there. Daily, I had to remind myself that if the prize was to be a restored immune system, what did a couple of years out of my life matter? After all, it had taken more years than that for my health to break down.

I still looked forward to the coffee breaks, except on days when I was too sick to read and could only lie on the bathroom floor, wishing for death. Sometimes, as I crawled from my bed to the bathroom, it seemed the therapy's sole purpose was to destroy my dignity and reduce my ego to ashes. All the things I was spared as a child—enemas, castor oil, preoccupation with the body's least elegant functions—were now a part of my daily life. More than ever I was grateful to have been raised in a religion that saved me from the many drugs and vaccines that are pumped so promiscuously into children today. Had I been given a fraction of these when young, my immune system would have collapsed when I was twenty instead of forty.

At times, it frightened me to realize how alone I was in this venture—like a rookie pilot flying solo over uncharted territory, aware that if I crashed there was no hope of rescue or survival. I didn't like to bother Beata too often with questions, for she had her own busy life to lead, and besides, our problems were not the same.

The only person to whom I could turn when faith was faltering was Charlotte, but she was a continent away and not always available. At such times I would listen to one of the tapes we recorded in my room or a talk she had given at a cancer convention. As Beata predicted, the mere sound of that strong, confident voice was enough to put the starch back in my spine and renew resolve.

There were times when, had it not been for Charlotte's voice at the end of the line, I might not have had the will to go on. She gave me hope and perspective on moonless nights. She was my long-distance cheerleader, my angel in absentia—my lifeline to recovery.

CHAPTER TWENTY-EIGHT

It was night in the lonesome October
Of my most immemorial year.
　　　　　　—Edgar Allen Poe

October was a month of unremitting pain. Arthritis flared in every joint and aches in every muscle. When I woke, my fingers were so stiff I could hardly close them around a pen and when I turned my head to the right, my neck felt like a column of splintered glass.

Again, I reached for the primer and turned to the chapter on healing reactions:

> During the reaction, arthritic joints may become puffed up and more painful than previously experienced.

An understatement, but a reassuring one. How perverse, I reflected, that we should draw comfort from knowing that others before us have suffered in the same distressing way.

On the 4th of October, I threw away all the antigen vaccines as an act of faith in the path I had chosen. It was an extravagant gesture for they were expensive and had hardly been used, but it seemed important to affirm my total reliance on the therapy.

Beata rang on the 5th to ask how I was getting on. After moaning to her about the arthritis, I moaned about my vanishing hair. I had already described its odd behavior that last night at the clinic and its subsequent collapse on the plane.

"And now," I wailed, "it's gone all limp again!"

"That's not possible," she said. "Hair is dead. It can't change. Its only life is in the roots."

"I know that, Beata. I can't understand either why mine behaves the way it does—curling one day and collapsing the next—but it's getting worse. Do you think this means it's a flare-up and therefore a good sign?"

"Well, everyone I know who has been on the therapy, their hair has got better, not worse, so I'm afraid it's not a very good sign."

Trust Beata to cheer me up, I thought. If only she weren't so honest.

Isilda's pep talks were worse. Each time I bewailed my thinning thatch she said, "My hair, too, it go like that! Always change when I am nair-voos and upset!"

"But I'm only nervous and upset *because* my hair is falling out!" I cried. Why could no one understand how maddening it was to be told, "I wouldn't worry, I think your hair looks fine," when you knew how it *should* look, and wanted to scream, "Well you jolly well *would* worry if it was *your* hair falling out and no one could tell you why!" Only the fact that I had so much hair to begin with kept friends from noticing its slow, backward slide.

By mid-October, most of my former allergies had returned. When I asked Beata what she thought this meant, she confessed she didn't know. "No one I know has had your problem," she explained. And that was my problem. None of the Gerson patients we knew had chemical poisoning, only cancer—although, increasingly, I suspected a link between the two.

Other flare-ups followed. Walking home from Kensington High Street tube station one day, I suddenly doubled up with stabbing pains in the groin. When I managed to reach my flat, I picked up the phone and called Charlotte, too worried to wait for a letter to creep through the transatlantic post.

"That's great!" she exclaimed. "A good sign the liver is beginning to get rid of its poisons. Are you taking the liver juice? No? You must try to get the baby calves' liver there— it hastens the healing." I groaned. "Only fresh young livers weighing not more than three or four pounds should be used," she cautioned. "These will not yet have been fed the hormones and steroids given to cows. Any nonorganic liver above that weight is certain to be contaminated."

I found a supplier and added three liver juices to the regime, replacing two carrots and a green. This brought predictable howls from Isilda, who hated change—even though *she* had been changing, from bossy but helpful to stroppy and despotic.

"At least you don't have to drink the stuff," I said, fishing for a crumb of sympathy.

"This liver," she retorted, "I like better drink than to make! My God, is hard to grind! And the juice cloths is *more* hard to clean! I tell you this," she warned, shaking a carrot at me, "this animal juice—it make you *more* sick!"

Having twigged by now that I was a wimp, Isilda began to exploit my dependence upon her in earnest. Perhaps the juices were stressing her out, I reasoned, or perhaps too much praise had gone to her head. If I said something she could construe as remotely critical she would shrug and say, "I do my best"—or, more pointedly, "You no like, I go!"

Easily intimidated, and too weak to stand up to her blackmail, I resorted to craven appeasement, which only made her worse. St. Paul got it wrong: The root of all evil is not the love of money—it's the love of *power!*[27]

Arriving at my desk with a juice, Isilda would plonk it down, point to my typewriter and command, "You put in your book that I go to *Heaven* for making all this juices! My God, what a job!"

And so—very meekly—I put in my book.

But she had been warned.

---

[27] First Epistle of St. Paul to Timothy.

As the days stretched into weeks and the weeks into months, I kept asking, *Why does my body so mightily betray me?* I had never abused it—never even been tempted by the things the young of today can scarcely avoid, yet it was full of rebellion.

Gerson warns that cancer flare-ups can last from two to four days and Beata recorded a total of twenty-eight flare-ups when she did the therapy. Being an arithmaphobe, I didn't even try to count mine, but there were headaches and muscle weakness and devastating fatigue and days of such constant sneezing that I seemed to be allergic to the universe. There was frustration with the functions that kept me body-bound and fury when the regime's demands ate into my time for work. There was loneliness and doubt and fear that it might not work for me—that the map I was given to follow had been charted for a different journey.

"My, what a lot of Karma you must be working through!" remarked a new-age friend, who had been following the therapy's ups and downs.

"Karma or chemicals," I retorted, "it is not a fun journey." Augusto Roa Bastos describes it best in *I, the Supreme:*

> I journeyed through all those great re-
> motenesses with only my own person at my
> side, without anybody. Alone. Without fam-
> ily. Alone. Without anybody. Alone in a
> strange country, the strangest one being that
> most my own. Alone. My trapped, lonely,
> alien country. Deserted. Alone. Full of my
> empty person.

Spot-on, Augusto.

And then there was depression—a full month of it. But I had a lot to be depressed about: becoming bald, ending the therapy more sensitive than when I began, mistaking a terminal crisis for a healing flare-up and so on. Frye warned us that depression was part of the healing process; he just forgot to add that it could be suicidal.

Thoughts of easeful death tempted many a midnight hour, my only restraint being the fear of opting out of life before its purpose had been fulfilled, assuming it had one. But what was I saving my life for? I had achieved nothing, would never finish my book, would be missed by no one if I died (this last, perhaps, a shade self-dramatizing).

There were times when I felt I couldn't go on, yet neither could I go back. *You've come this far,* I kept telling myself. *You can't give up now. But how long, oh, Lord, how long?*

To my diary, one night, I whined:

> Dear God, have I been struggling to save
> my life, only to die—not in a paroxysm of
> pain, but in a whimper of despair?

To this whimper of self-pity there came only silence. Divine neglect, not divine punishment, is the worst.

At times, the only thing that kept me going was false hope—hope that my daughters still needed me, that torments such as these afflict only the virtuous and so forth. Most of what sustains us in life is illusion, but is no less sustaining for that.

The word "courage" was much on my mind at this time—chiefly because of its irrelevance when faced with a challenge that can't be escaped. To be courageous requires an element of volition, with the option *not* to be courageous—such as taking the bullet in battle to save a comrade's life, or rescuing a drowning child when one hardly knows how to swim. Enduring what can't be changed isn't courage; it's fortitude.

Toward the end of October the arthritic flare-ups grew milder, which suggested to me that some forms of arthritis may be caused by a settling of toxins in the joints. If this is so, then the stiffening joint should be viewed as a warning to detoxify the body—not as a sign to relieve the symptoms with more chemicals in the form of drugs.

On the 25th of October, I woke at 4:30 in the morning with my neck feeling like a block of crystal being crushed by a wrench. Pains shot through my legs and the soles of my feet felt as if they were plugged into a low-voltage electric socket. It was my strongest flare-up to date and the scariest. To be facing this crisis armed only with juices and enemas made me feel like a very small David confronting Goliath with an organic carrot. This Goliath, however, was a monster of many parts, all of them man-made and all of them lethal.

I staggered into the bathroom and glanced in the mirror, only to recoil in horror from the image I saw staring back at me. The distorted features, the inflamed patches under my eyes and the wisps of hair flying away from my head—it was as if I had morphed into some alien creature.

My mind flew back to the end of World War II and the family friend who contracted a mysterious disease while serving in the Pacific theatre. Young and handsome when he left for the war, his features began to change even before he was discharged. His hair fell out, his strong body wasted away and he grew prematurely old before our eyes. When he died in his thirties, leaving a wife and young children, he was almost unrecognizable.

"Something he caught in the Pacific," the family said, but no one really knew.

Fortunately, my features returned to normal within a few hours. All the same, the incident gave me pause. Could the erosion of that young soldier's body have been caused by some unknown chemical he was exposed to even then? I had met a Vietnam War veteran who attributed the birth of an albino son, conceived after his return home, to his known exposure to Agent Orange. And I met a group of Gulf War veterans whose afflictions were so manifestly caused by chemical poisoning, they should silence forever those who deny the reality of Gulf War Syndrome.

Perhaps the war to end all wars is the one being waged even now within our bodies—between the toxins whose

196

ever-increasing number we can neither know nor prevent, yet the cumulative power of which may one day bring us all down in defeat.

CHAPTER TWENTY-NINE

Tumbling and tumbling I aspired to heaven.
—Philip Toynbee

November brought a letter from Nora telling me of David's death.

"Even though it was expected," she wrote, "I'm still feeling devastated by his loss."

How hard it is, I reflected, when we are the ones left behind, to believe that death is merely a change of worlds. Whatever view we may hold of the hereafter, life still unfolds in a veil of mystery.

On the 4th of November, my mastectomy scar developed a pinkish aura and began to itch. Fascinated, I watched the area grow red and become engorged. Could I be growing a new breast? Alas, the therapy doesn't restore missing bits. After five days the swelling and inflammation subsided, leaving me in awe of the body's ability to tidy up the debris of an eleven-year-old operation.

I recalled my oncologist saying he wished all his patients were as easy as I was. At the time, I took this to be a compliment. Now, however, I knew that being easy, being compliant, was precisely what I should *not* have been. I had yielded to the knife as trustingly as I yielded to prayer, when what I should have done was rage, rebel, and refuse to be butchered. At least I had the sense to reject the hysterectomy he wanted to perform—"to prevent your crazy hormones from creating cancer in the other breast," he explained. I had heard enough hysterectomy horror stories to know that when the time came, I wanted my menopause to be a natural one.

I thought of the so-called "cancer-prone personality" theory, suggested by Lawrence LeShan, whose books I was then reading. "Emotionally repressed" and "unable to express love or aggression" were two of the characteristics ascribed to such individuals. It was true that I found it hard to express aggression, but emotionally repressed? Unable to express love? Hardly. In my view, the emotional-traits-as-cause-of-disease theory comes close to blaming the victim again. Even Beata favored the psychological approach— understandably so, for by then she was a practicing psychotherapist.

One day, when we were discussing our different cancers, Beata proposed an exercise:

"Try to identify the psychological factors that might have contributed to the development of your breast cancer," she suggested.

I tried to do this, but could not honestly see a connection between my psyche and a tumor. Even if there was one, what useful purpose could be served by identifying it? After all, we can't change our basic personalities. A more likely factor, it seemed to me, was the smoke from my father's cigars, which filled my girlhood home with a carcinogenic smog.

Not that I denied the mind/body/spirit connection. How could I, when members of my family and I had experienced numerous healings in Christian Science? It was simply that I knew people who fit the psychological model for cancer, yet whom it had never touched, while others, who could not have been more different, succumbed to the disease. Theory aside, whatever psychological factors may have contributed to Beata's cancer, it was the body-bound Gerson Therapy that cured her melanoma.

By November 10th, I was detoxing so fast my body resembled a medical repertory company: *EACH DAY A NEW FLARE-UP! EACH WEEK A NEW CAST OF SYMPTOMS!* Some flare-ups were so strong I needed an extra juice during the intermission (I'd have settled for an intermission). If a crisis arose during the night I added an extra coffee break to speed the toxins on their way. During one break, I was so exhausted I fell asleep on the bathroom floor—waking to find myself with a hose stuck up my bottom and a nasty crick in my neck. "Why you no wake me?" demanded Isilda the next morning, all noisy commiseration when she learned I'd been ill during the night.

Bewildered by the multiplicity of symptoms, I wrote to Charlotte:

> What do they mean, these random pains throughout my body—these hot flushes one moment, chills the next and legs so weak I have to drag myself up the stairs?

Her reply arrived on the 13th of November:

> We see that in patients who have old drug damage. We always get a different reaction from the cancer patient, who usually hasn't been as totally pre-treated with drugs, unless they've had chemo. The drug damage and healing are rough.

So that was all right, then; things were coming along nicely.

Seizing this small comfort, I soldiered on through an attack of cystitis that mimicked one I'd had thirteen years earlier, along with rashes that broke out on different parts of my body, the one on my fingers having since healed. My swollen toe, too, had returned to normal. As for the calluses on my feet, they were so nearly gone I could almost forget about them during the day.

Isilda, meanwhile, who had a soft spot beneath her crusty exterior, came into my room one morning with a book in her hand.

"I like you read this book," she said. "If you do, it make you better." A glance at the cover told me it was the

Christian Science textbook, *Science and Health, with Key to the Scriptures,* by Mary Baker Eddy. "My friend," explained Isilda, "she take me to Wednesday night meeting and I like very much. She give me tapes of sermons. I tell you, God will heal you if you read this book."

There was something endearing about the Catholic Isilda urging me to turn for healing to the Protestant faith I had relinquished years before. Deeply moved, I thanked her for her concern, adding that I already had the book and would read it again at the earliest opportunity.

By mid-November, there were days when I was feeling almost well—well enough to attend to the chores I had neglected when too ill to function. Remissions, however, were short-lived. As soon as toxins entered my bloodstream again, the parade of flare-ups resumed its merry round.

Dear God, get me through the night! was a frequent entry in my diary at this time. But what was I keeping a diary for? With no secrets to confide, no juicy scandals to record, it was just a tedious account of symptoms, fears and moans.

On the 17th of November, I felt an odd pressure in my lungs, similar to the one I experienced the day Clive left a Malachite stone on my map. I called him to ask if a similar accident had occurred.

"No," he said. "As a matter of fact, the last time this happened I decided to keep your map in a manila envelope to protect it from the others in the room, so whatever is bothering you, it must be something in your flat."

What, then, could it be? Isilda was off that day, and I had made only two juices. How anyone could do the therapy on their own, especially when having a flare-up, was beyond me; yet I was told that a few plucky patients had done just that—and successfully, too.

I was in the kitchen that evening when Isilda returned around ten. As I went to greet her, I caught a whiff of perfume on her person. This surprised me, for she had agreed not to use any scented products while staying in the flat. In exchange for her compliance, I kept her supplied with fragrance-free soap, hand lotion, and shampoo.

"Isilda," I asked, "are you wearing perfume?"

"I no wear perfume since I come here!" she said, crossly, unwinding the scarf from around her neck.

"But I can smell it. There's some sort of scent on your body."

"All I do—I put hair spray before I go out, that is all."

So that was it! The propellant in hair spray is one of the most volatile chemical pollutants there are. Isilda turned to go to her room, but I caught her arm.

"Wait, Isilda, I know this is hard for you to understand, but for someone who is chemically sensitive, *any* scented product—even hair spray—can be as troublesome as perfume."

"But I put on and go right out!" she insisted, her face darkening.

"I understand that, but you see—while *you* may have gone out, your hair spray stayed behind in the form of chlorofluorocarbons in the air."

She gave me a look of withering scorn. Isilda had no time for talk of chemicals or allergies, which she viewed as inventions of my addled brain. Yet she told me once that whenever she came near a fly she broke out in a rash. This seemed to me much odder than reacting to perfume. One day, however, when a fly gained entry to the flat—how, I shall never know—Isilda did indeed develop a rash, even before she was aware of the intruder's presence. Like it or not, Isilda was every bit as freakish as I. Together, we proved that, although you can fool the mind some of the time, you can't fool the body—at least, not for long.

Because of the large quantity of vegetables the therapy required—far more than I could carry home alone—I took Isilda with me when I went to the greengrocer for our weekly supply. Striding ahead of me on the pavement, her arms swinging like a drill sergeant's, while I trailed along behind her like an untouchable, she cut a singular figure.

Even poor Mr. Desai was not spared the sharp end of her tongue, her caustic comments about his blameless produce making me cringe with embarrassment. On one occasion, after she flounced out of the store while I was paying the bill, his dark eyes followed her retreating figure before returning to meet mine.

"How do you put up with her?" he asked, shaking his head.

"With difficulty," I replied.

Three months into the therapy, on the morning of November 27th, I woke at 3:00 a.m. with a socking headache, a feeling of nausea and renewed stiffness in my legs. The usual detox measures having failed, I turned for reassurance to the primer's chapter on healing reactions:

> . . . Lack of appetite, nausea, headache, arthritic symptoms, flu-like aches in the body . . . .

Marginally less alarmed, I spent the day in bed nursing my pounding head, while ignoring Isilda's demands that I quit the therapy.

That evening, as I was releasing an enema, a searing fire shot through my rectum. It was though a hot poker was thrust up my backside. The pain could not have lasted more than sixty seconds, but it was so excruciating I cried out in agony. When the burning stopped I searched the bowl for some evidence of the cause, but there was none. However, the greenish color of the return told me that a strong detox phase was underway. No wonder Gerson patients say, "If you can survive the therapy, you can survive anything."

In less than an hour my headache lifted and the nausea was gone. The next morning, I was able to sit cross-legged on the floor when meditating for the first time in weeks. It was a flaming miracle! As the Buddha said, "One of the signs of fire is change."

But how could my body have harbored such a burning substance unawares—perhaps even for years? Was that the chemical I sometimes felt creeping under my scalp, destroying my eyebrows and eyelashes too? Had I poisoned the hair follicles by dyeing my hair a more lively auburn? Charlotte warns cancer patients against dyeing their hair. Oh, Charlotte, where were you when I was foolish and twenty? Where were you when I was foolish and forty!

Baffled by the burning backside incident, I rang Beata to ask if something similar had happened to her when she was doing the therapy.

"Not quite," she said, "but I once woke up with a bilious burning sensation in my mouth."

No wonder doctors scoffed at the idea of chemical sensitivity. What self-respecting physician would link a rectum on fire with pesticide poisoning or a bilious burning sensation in the mouth with melanoma die-off? Chemicals don't show up on X-rays or conventional tests. One has to know what to look for—and where, and how.

As evidence grew that my psychosomatic illness had a very somatic cause, so did my gratitude to Charlotte for keeping the flame of her father's work alive. How different the face of medicine might be today had Gerson received in this country the recognition he was on the verge of receiving in his own. How different my own fate might have been, were it not for a friend whose life his therapy had saved.

I wish I could say that I never lost faith, but I did; that in the darkest moments I knew I would be healed, but I didn't. Doubt was never further away than the next flare-up and each time despair got a hold on my spirit, the only thing that kept me from giving up was—well, giving up.

Sometimes I felt like that child who, when ill, ran to her mother's room at night, wondering if the sudden fever or mindless panic really was just a "belief" that could be healed by prayer. More often than not it was, but when it wasn't, Mother called a Christian Science practitioner to give me "absent treatment." It was probably as well for the practitioner—and for me—that I was born an exceptionally healthy and resilient child.

Looking back on those nights, my strongest memory is not of any particular illness, for none were diagnosed, but of the spiritual confusion they engendered. Secretly, I feared that if I should ever be faced with a life-or-death crisis, my faith would not be strong enough to prevail. And if faith should fail? Beyond Christian Science lay a scary world of doctors and hospitals—the only Satans in our sunny, optimistic religion. And because that world was unknown and its arts forbidden, the thought that I might have to turn to it one day filled me with fear.

I had reached my thirties when the crisis occurred. Had it not brought me close to death, I doubt that anything could have torn me from my faith or forced me to examine more deeply the roots of my religion. Now, forty years on, and with the only person I could turn to for help a world away, it seemed as though long-distance healing had been woven into the fabric of my life—perhaps even before I was born.

CHAPTER THIRTY

. . . Love your solitude and bear with sweet-sounding
lamentation the suffering it causes you.
—Rainer Maria Rilke

In December, the black dog of depression returned, dragging me down below the surface of life to a dark and desolate place. I should have realized that this, too, was part of the detoxification process, for pesticides poison the brain as well as the body. Yet reason vanishes when a voice inside one's head keeps saying, *What is the use? What is it all for?*

When I thought of the years of self-denial that lay ahead my discouragement deepened, for I knew it would take more than eighteen months to rid my body of its chemical burden. Why shouldn't it take years to shed what had taken half a lifetime to acquire?

How much of what kept me going was faith and how much sheer doggedness, I cannot say. Part of what sustained me when days were darkest was the feeling there must be others going through a similar experience, who were just as bewildered and discouraged as I.

Lurching from flare-up to flare-up, from chronic fatigue symptoms to flu-like fevers to aches of bewildering origin, I kept asking the question every sufferer has asked since the dawn of time: *Why me? Why this?* The only answer that came was the one a guard at Auschwitz is said to have given a doomed inmate: *"Hier gibt es kein warum."* "Here there is no why."

There were nights when self-pity scratched at the soul and I longed for the touch of a human hand in the dark. Tony was dying of liver and colon cancer, but had to stop chemotherapy because it made him so ill. He, too, needed a comforting presence now, far more than did I. But just when our mutual need was greatest, neither was able to comfort the other. Wondering why life's testing times seemed always to come when I was alone, I consoled myself with the thought that at least I wasn't burdening a husband or lover with my illness. How many relationships could survive the therapy's romance-destroying, detumescing demands?

One day in December, while releasing an enema, I passed what appeared to be a long piece of string. Wondering how such an object could have entered my body, on closer inspection I realized it must be a worm. Stupidly, I seized a plastic comb and tried to retrieve it with the handle, but it kept sliding off so I gave up. That I could be harboring parasites would not have surprised me, for with my husband I had traveled extensively in Greece, Yugoslavia and the Middle East—countries where parasites are prevalent.

In 1979, I was sent to a well-known parasitologist in New York who confirmed the presence of giardia and amoebae in my gut. He even let me peer through his microscope to see what the amoeba looked like. A small, roundish thing, it resembled a transparent potato and would have been invisible when excreted. I could only assume that my worm met a nasty end during one of my chemical flare-ups, for given the rich nutritional environment I was providing, no sensible worm would have wanted to leave.

By mid-December, the toxins must have reached my brain, for I was in a state that can only be described as semi-deranged. One moment I was yearning for flare-ups as proofs of progress—then, when they came, fearing they were proofs of defeat. And defeat seemed imminent the day I rang Charlotte with a litany of despair.

"...And even my grip on reality seems to be weakening, Charlotte," I concluded.

"But that's *fine!*" she exclaimed. "You're right on schedule, having completed your fourth month. How often are you taking the castor oil? Only once a week? Make it twice for a while."

Aaargh! Oh, well, what doesn't kill me makes me stronger.

Or sicker.

As the weeks dragged by I began to chafe at the social restraints the therapy imposed. Friends could visit, of course, and I could visit them, taking my juice in a thermos, but the carefree pleasures I took for granted were a thing of the past. Gone were weekend seminars in the country, cozy dinners in ethnic restaurants, attending a play, ignoring the hour. Would I ever again know moments of sheer light-hearted fun?

What compelled adherence to such a socially limiting discipline? With no pills to take, no doctor to see, and no one to check that I didn't cheat, the only one to lose if I did cheat would be me.

Bored with my world's diminishing horizons, I decided to throw Gerson to the wind one evening and have a few friends in to dinner. Surely four months of self-denial deserved one night of shame-free self-indulgence.

"Guess what, Isilda?" I announced, cornering her in the kitchen. "We're going to have a dinner party! What do you think of that?"

She looked up from the chopping board with a scowl.

"What? You make your friends eat this food-with-no-taste?"

"Of course not," I laughed, pinching a leaf of romaine to chew on while having a think. "It will be a proper meal, with wine and cheese and . . . let's see, perhaps a ratatouille."

"A what?"

"It's a vegetable dish. Don't worry, I'll help you make it. Of course, not all the vegetables will be organic, but it shouldn't matter just this once."

"You no give your friends this juices," she warned, beheading a carrot with a vigorous chop. "I no make extra juices!"

"I wouldn't dream of it," I assured her.

In the event, the dinner was delicious, the company convivial, and the headache I woke up with the next morning was a beaut. *It's not fair!* I wailed to an unforgiving God. *I didn't even touch the wine!*

Around this time it dawned on me that I hadn't craved a piece of chocolate or a potato chip since the therapy began; but then where would such cravings find room in a stomach awash with juice? Of course, if someone placed a box of chocolates in front of me and left the room, I could not have vouched for my self-restraint, but the addictive element—that craving at odd hours of the day or night—was gone. This seemed to me as remarkable as the shrinking of a tumor or Beata's release from a thirty-year nicotine addiction. Perhaps my days of cowering before telluric energies also now were numbered.

I was anticipating this happy prospect when a friend came to dinner on Christmas Eve and again I abandoned my diet. Shortly after retiring, that sickly tide in the head returned. Had it been pain I could have taken a pill, but there were no drugs for this internal anarchy—no way to turn it off when it became unbearable. What can you do when you feel you are losing your mind? Where can you go when you want to jump out of your skin?

It took more faith than I could muster that night to believe that by the end of 1986 I would be much nearer recovery. Sleepless and depressed, I wandered to the window and stared into the darkness. The night was without a star. Where in that clouded heaven was the light to guide me? Where, the King of Peace? Hiding, both of them—like that old man on the mountaintop.

No star. No peace. No guide. Only endless, unremitting night.

CHAPTER THIRTY-ONE

I learn it daily, learn it with pain to which
I am grateful; patience is everything!
—Rainer Maria Rilke

In January of '86, I came upon a book called, *When the Snakes Awake,* about the changes in animal behavior that occur before an earthquake. Earthquakes being of singular interest to Californians, the ability of animals to sense them in advance intrigued me. The author, Helmut Tributsch—a professor of physical chemistry in Berlin at the time—had culled reports from many countries of anomalous animal behavior that occurred hours and even days before an earthquake.

Noting that well-water levels can change before a quake, the water becoming cloudy or discolored, he concludes that some sort of geophysical process takes place in the ground before a quake, which sensitive animals pick up in advance.[28]

In one section, titled "Human Earthquake Premonition," an Italian scientist describes the physiological reactions certain people experienced prior to an earthquake that shook the Italian province of Piedmont in 1808:

> The more nervous people were seized, for
> some time before the tremors, by a certain

---

[28] Before the Indian Ocean tsunami on Dec. 26, 2004, most of the animals, especially the elephants, fled to higher ground.

inexplicable restlessness, by a kind of trembling and pounding of the heart.

As I read this, I felt a sudden click of recognition. That last night at the clinic . . . my pounding heart and trembling feet . . . . could they have been premonitory symptoms of the quake that was to rock Mexico City thirty-eight hours later? The very idea was absurd. And yet, the experience of a writer who lived through a severe earthquake in Copiapo, Chile, in 1822, sounded eerily familiar. Describing the disaster signal as "an inexplicable condition of the nervous system that manifests itself before any other sign of the earthquake," he continues:

> Before we hear the sound, or at least are fully conscious of hearing it, we are made sensible, I do not know how, that something uncommon is going to happen; everything seems to change color; our thoughts are chained immovably down; the whole world appears to be in disorder; all nature looks different to what it is wont to do; and we feel quite subdued and overwhelmed by some invisible power, beyond human control or apprehension.

These words described so vividly my experience that night—even to the disordered earth energies my rod and color wheel revealed—that I read on with mounting interest.

> During a severe earthquake, the sensations of sensitive people escalate greatly. . . Certain people whose health has been undermined by illness or addiction seem to be extraordinarily sensitive to an approaching earthquake.

People whose health has been undermined by illness . . . Could my illness, then, have rendered me extraordinarily sensitive to the impending disaster? According to Tributsch, the average time span between an observed behavior anomaly and an earthquake can be from two hours to two days. How strong the quake must be, or how near the person to its epicenter, he doesn't say. The Mexico City quake registered a staggering 8.1 on the Richter scale, but the clinic was almost 1,500 miles away.[29]

Risible though such speculation may be, it did not seem unreasonable to ask: If animals can sense an impending change in the earth hours, or even days before an earthquake, why shouldn't human beings sense it as well? Perhaps we did in the past when we were more in tune with the earth and its rhythms, before the distractions of civilization deadened our senses to the subtler whisperings of nature.

As for the renascence of my hair the following morning—could that, too, have been a harbinger of the quake to come? If we assume hair to be analogous to a growing plant, a clue may be found in a report of the Peking Geological Bureau concerning an earthquake that occurred in 1971 near the Yangtze River. Under the heading, "Do plants have reactions before earthquakes?" the report described how "flowers, shrubs, and trees bloomed in winter as harbingers of terror, death, and destruction."

In three different provinces, prior to three earthquakes in different years, potato vines, yarrow plants, and Chinese cabbage bloomed out of season weeks before the event. In Haicheng province, apricot trees flowered in winter two months before the February 4th quake in 1975.

Referring to these anomalies, Tributsch comments:

> These types of examples do not seem too nu-
> merous, and very few people mention them.
> Actually, some plants do have anomalous re-

---

[29] A commission that investigated the California quake of April 18, 1906, found that adverse effects on human health were most frequent in the border areas of the earthquake zone, where the earth's movements had been rather weak.

actions before earthquakes ... It may be that in the rest of the world similar phenomena are simply not acknowledged because the observers lack sophistication and because the catastrophe does not happen.

Had I not chanced upon this book, it would not have occurred to me to link my body's behavior that night with the earthquake that devastated Mexico City a day and a half later. And had it not been for my modest dowsing skill, I would not have known that my bewildering symptoms were being caused by a massive change in the environment.

Why, then, did these symptoms grow weaker as we drove to Los Angeles the next day? Maybe it was because I was moving away from the epicenter of the coming quake. Or perhaps my body needed to be earthed—connected to the ground in some way—in order to sense the vibrations.

Intriguing though these speculations were, without some way of proving them they would remain mere conjecture. I was unlikely to find myself in the same situation again—nor had I any wish to repeat the experience. Since proof was impossible, I consigned the incident to that growing file labeled "mysterious occurrences," and turned my thoughts to more immediate concerns.

And there the subject would have remained, had not my visit home that December coincided with what I can only describe as a timely gift from Mother Nature.

CHAPTER THIRTY-TWO

*I now recognize that with each discovery
the extent of the unknown grows larger,
not smaller.*

—James Lovelock

The New Year began in much the same way as the old with morning headaches, waves of sickness, and hair that clung to my scalp like wet fur on a dog's back. Why linger longer on this planet, I reasoned, when so much of what I cherished has been polluted or destroyed?

Isilda, too, was growing more disobliging by the day, her small eyes narrowing more often, her peasant hands crossing more defiantly over her apron to denote disapproval. Silent and sullen, she marched ahead of me on the way to the greengrocer, asserting her dominance by the distance she put between us.

No week went by without her moans about the juices, and lately she'd been getting the sequence wrong—like an actor in a long-running play who grows bored and begins to forget his lines. She, however, could leave in September—or tomorrow, as she kept reminding me—whereas I was stuck with an indefinite run.

Quite simply, Isilda needed a change—and so did I.

On the last day of February, 1986, Tony died. He was only fifty-seven, a lover of literature and an organizer of regional concerts for London's symphony orchestras. We had shared operas at Glyndebourne, concerts in cathedrals, and unforgettable evenings at Covent Garden. For fifteen years he filled my life with love, laughter, and music, and now he was gone—leaving behind a void that could never again be filled in the same inspiriting way.

In the seventh month of the therapy, I experienced a return of that mini-generator operating under my skin. Alarmed at this apparent setback, I rang Charlotte.

"From what you tell me of your symptoms," she said, "you may be detoxifying too fast. I suggest you reduce the juices to six." (Isilda *will* be pleased.) "But don't be too tied down to the intensive therapy," she warned. "Do what your body tells you to do."

"But my body keeps telling me it hasn't a clue, Charlotte."

A pause. "Have you taken much Valium in the past?"

"Yes . . . although not since my divorce. I was taking three a day before, with two sleeping pills at night, but the only Valium I've had since is the tranquillizer they give you before an operation, which I don't need."

"Tranquillizers are much harder to get rid of than chemicals," said Charlotte. "Psychotropic drugs stay in the body for years, but doctors never diagnose Valium poisoning because it can't be detected. Anyway, few of them even believe it exists. The benzodiazepines and antidepressants will cause burning and hot flushes and loss of hair."

Could that fire in the rectum, then, have been caused by Valium I hadn't taken for years? The flushes and hair loss too? If it was interacting with other drugs in my body, there was no telling how nasty a brew had evolved, the chemical whole being more lethal than the sum of its toxic parts.

Isilda reduced the juices accordingly, but it was the end of April before I was able to sleep comfortably again in my bed. By then, there were even days when I felt almost well. It was this paradox of feeling normal one moment and ghastly the next that made environmental illness so difficult for doctors to take seriously, and so easy for the unknowing to dismiss.

215

On the 28th of April, a disaster occurred in the Soviet Union when a nuclear reactor at Chernobyl raged out of control. The first radioactive clouds arrived over Britain on the first of May, accompanied by the usual government assurances: "The levels are too low to present any danger!" How could they tell? By the time the full danger is known, there may be no one left to lie to.

One morning in June, I woke with a sharp pain in my right buttock. Having learned that new pains can refer to old injuries, I cast my mind back and recalled a minor skiing accident in France in 1983. While clutching the T-bar of the ski lift pulling us up the mountain, I became so entranced with the scenery I forgot to let go when the lift reached the landing station. Only when my skis left the ground and I saw the empty bars ahead of me swinging over a deep valley, did I come to my senses in time to let go.

The drop to the ground could not have been more than eight feet, but the sharp landing on my right hip put paid to the rest of my skiing holiday. As with previous flare-ups, the pain in my buttock subsided within a week.

Also in June, Isilda's moods were beginning to grate. Each Iberian oath that issued from the kitchen, each "you-no-like-I-go" ultimatum, made me long for a placid, monosyllabic Swede as her replacement. No governess of my childhood (it was that kind of childhood) was more domineering—not even the termagant who washed my mouth out with soap for some childish oath and locked me in a closet as dark as an Egyptian tomb, thus spawning a lifelong claustrophobia.

As my health improved the flare-ups were fewer, but in the forty-second week of the therapy I had the sort of migraine attack that made me glad Isilda was off that day, so I could suffer in peace. Her growing truculence, coupled with Tony's death and my distant daughters, neither of whom were inclined to pick up a telephone or employ a pen, added to my sense of abandonment by the few people I needed most in my life.

I was at my lowest ebb when an incident occurred that struck such despair in my heart, it sent me hurtling over the edge into a mindless fury. The anger flare-up had been long in coming, but when it came it hit me with a wallop. Rage I had suppressed for a lifetime erupted with a frenzy I was helpless to control. Every mistake I had ever made—each foolish, stupid, gullible thing I had said or done—exploded in my brain with the J'accuse of an avenging angel.

Seizing a large cushion from the sofa I began to pummel it with my fists, hurling blows upon my father whose bullying I blamed for turning me into a wimp, and beating the hell out of that scorpion self that was forever stinging me with its tail. When I wanted to sleep my anger kept me awake and when I woke it was still there—pounding away in my brain like a remorseless fever. I wanted to weep, curse, howl, shake my fist at heaven, strike out at anything and *everything* that was turning my world upside down, and all I could do was beat the stuffing out of an innocent pillow.

Even in my unhinged state I remembered my arrogant assumption that *I* would not be prey to the kind of anger flare-up Beata had experienced. Yet here I was, stomping all over her well-trodden footsteps like a beastly child, behaving as badly as she did and being ashamed of myself into the bargain.

For days I functioned on the periphery of amnesia, forgetting appointments, losing a thought in mid-sentence and losing my short-term memory altogether. Like an empty train hurtling toward disaster, I was manifesting all the signs of toxic psychosis.

Tooling along Brompton road in the wrong direction one day, I mistook the row of cars on my left for being parked instead of waiting for the light to change. When I realized my mistake it was as if I'd been jolted out of a trance. As the cars began to move forward, I made a U-turn and squeezed into the queue—right in front of a police car, which promptly flashed its lights at me to pull over.

Cringing with shame, I watched in the side-view mirror as a young officer got out of his car and walked up to my window.

"Are you aware, madam," he asked, with pained courtesy, "that you were in the lane for oncoming cars and were therefore creating a traffic hazard?"

"I know . . . I mean, no." I stammered. "I didn't realize . . . that is, I'm sorry, officer, but I've been ill and I'm afraid I haven't been thinking clearly."

"Do you think you should be driving in this condition?" he asked, not unkindly.

"I don't think I should be *living* in this condition," I replied.

The officer must have had a soft heart, for he let me off with only a caution. All the same, the incident was so worrying that I rang Charlotte.

"A *very* good sign!" she exclaimed. "Normally, anger doesn't surface until the main part of the healing has been gone through. In most cases, the chemicals in the brain are the last to mobilize into the bloodstream."

Try telling that to the policeman, I wanted to say, or to the people I alienated while the balance of my mind was disturbed. Fortunately, my anger petered out from sheer exhaustion, and by the first of July I regained some measure of equanimity.

With Isilda's departure imminent in September, I began to search for her replacement in August.

"I think I've found someone, Isilda," I announced on the 21st. "She's a Polish lady, Bronya—late thirties, I think, and quite pleasant-seeming. I've invited her to come by tomorrow to watch you make a couple of juices, so she'll have some idea of the procedure when she begins."

"Why you invite?" Isilda demanded, irritably. "I no like she watch me when I work."

"Oh, come, come, it's only for an hour." As I might have foreseen, Isilda behaved so rudely to the young woman, replying curtly to her questions and making no effort to be helpful or even civil, that I had to make apologies to Bronya when saying good-bye to her at the door.

Returning to the kitchen, I gave vent to my new-found anger. "Really, Isilda, you might at least have *tried* to be polite," I said. But she affected not to hear. Turning away, she picked up the dishcloth and began to make a pointed show of cleaning the juicing machine.

Two weeks before she was to leave, on the night of August 22nd, Isilda came into the sitting room lugging the two suitcases she was sending ahead to Portugal.

"I bring for you to look before I send . . . see I no steal nothing."

"Steal?" I echoed. "Of course I won't look through your things, Isilda. What an idea! When have I ever questioned your honesty?"

She made no reply, but trundled the cases back to her room. Days later, after running an errand for me at the chemist's, she thrust her open palm at me with the change.

"Here, you count, see I do not steal."

"I will *not* count," I snapped. "What *is* all this about stealing, Isilda? You know I've never mistrusted you!"

As though trust was an added affront, her mouth tightened and she marched off to the kitchen, hands sweeping the sides of her apron in that gesture of irritation that I found amusing at first, but which now had me grinding my teeth. Could I endure fourteen more days of Isilda without closing my hands around her throat?

On the eve of her departure, she confronted me after dinner, the gimlet eyes narrowing.

"How much money you give me when I go?" she asked. "Four-week vacation, yes?"

Even after a year, Isilda's audacity could still astonish. Legally, there was no obligation to give her a penny, but four weeks was what I had planned. Being *ordered* to do so, however, was another matter. Anger loosened my reluctant tongue and I lost my temper.

"What makes you think I *wouldn't* do the right thing by you, Isilda?" I demanded. "Have I ever cheated you? Tell me, have I? Frankly, your attitude these past months has driven me round the bend and as for your complaints, I've had *those* right up to here! At times your behavior has been so . . . so *uncalled* for, it was all I could do to keep from telling you off!"

Stunned by this outburst, which took us both by surprise, Isilda for once was speechless. If only *I* had been as well, for even as the words left my lips I regretted them.

"Oh, forgive me, Isilda," I said, anger collapsing like a dud soufflé. "I've been under a strain lately . . . some personal problems and . . . well, it's just that you *could* have been more helpful at times." Seeing the storm clouds gather, I added, "I'm sorry. Please forgive me."

But Isilda, for whom a grievance was gold, was not about to forgive. Turning on her heel she swept wordlessly away, closing her bedroom door with an eloquent bang. Sick with remorse, I spent the night reproaching myself for my loss of control. How could I patch things up in the morning before she left?

The next day, I waited until Isilda had her suitcase in the hall before trying to slip the vacation money into her coat pocket, but she pushed my hand angrily away. Seizing her bags, she made for the door—pausing on the threshold only to deliver a parting shot:

"I think now, when I go . . . you fumigate my room, yes?"

As I watched her dark figure disappear down the stairs, I wondered if any part of my life made sense anymore. Was there something in me that brought out the madness in others, or was I even madder than I could bring myself to believe? I closed the door, reflecting with a leaden heart that these things must be sent to try us. No doubt Isilda found me as heavy a number to live with as I found her—although, in a funny way, I was going to miss her. She may have been difficult, but she was never dull.

When I think of her now, I see her sitting in a Portuguese piazza on a balmy summer's evening, enjoying her Bacalhau and Madeira, while entertaining friends with tales of "all this juices" she had to make for a crazy American, who was so crackers she kept putting coffee up her behind.

Ah, well, with luck, Isilda will never know that it worked.

CHAPTER THIRTY-THREE

We all look at Nature too much,
And live with her too little.
—Oscar Wilde

Bronya had been in situ only a week when the suspicion grew that I might have exchanged one kind of domestic demon for another. There was no hint at our interview of the manic carnivore who would fill the flat with the fumes of frying meat and make heavy weather of the simplest task. Slow and disorganized, she fussed over trifles while leaving important things undone—such as letting leafy vegetables wilt on the draining board instead of putting them in the refrigerator when no longer needed. Juices arrived erratically and dishes piled up in the sink until after dinner. Since she rarely finished before nine the chaos in the kitchen was chronic.

Too disheartened to look for someone else, I told myself not to be such a bloody perfectionist and tried to avert my eyes. Aspects of her behavior, however, led me to suspect that at some time in the past Bronya might have suffered a nervous breakdown. Disarmed initially by her soft voice and gentle manner, I soon discovered they cloaked a nature every bit as controlling as Isilda's. Four weeks into the job, she demanded an increase in the salary she had described as "generous" the day she was engaged.

At first, I attributed her mood swings to the premenstrual tension she warned me about, but there seemed to be no cyclical pattern to her compulsive-addictive behavior. If I entered the kitchen after dinner, I found her standing there with a dreamy, faraway look in her eyes, lovingly polishing a saucepan that already gleamed like a burnished jewel. Although we did our laundry separately, she refused to use the washing machine—"because," she explained, reproachfully, "you sometimes put your underpants in the same load with the sheets!"

Unable to feel much guilt about this, I dismissed her concern as just another of Bronya's little quirks. One day, however, after she had put my laundered clothes into the dryer, she approached my desk holding something aloft between her forefinger and thumb with an air of fastidious distaste.

"Look!" she cried, accusingly. *"Look* what I found in your laundry! A pubic hair!"

I sighed. "Well, at least it's a clean pubic hair," I observed, and went on with my work.

Although Bronya's need to control was subtler than Isilda's, it was not long before my inner wimp was caving in to her demands as well. What was it in me that brought out the bully in women? I wondered. Did I really need another dominatrix in my life?

In the course of my reading that fall, I came upon a reference to the HealthMed Detoxification Program in Los Angeles—a three- to four-week regime based on dry saunas and aerobic exercise. Conceived by the late L. Ron Hubbard of Scientology fame—presumably to detoxify those of his followers who were hooked on drugs—it reportedly was helping victims of environmental illness as well.

Like most Gerson patients, I wished there was an easier, less labor-intensive method of detoxifying the body that would still be as effective. I doubted, however, that a month of saunas could achieve anything like the same results. Then, too, I was leery of the Hubbard connection.

When I lived in Paris in the 1960s, an acquaintance gave me a copy of Hubbard's book, *Dianetics*, to read and invited me to a Scientology meeting. Having recently left the church

I was open to new ideas, but I found Hubbard's book so unreadable, and aspects of the movement so dubious, I was not surprised to learn that in his previous incarnation he had been a writer of science fiction. Was HealthMed a front for luring the addicted into the religion, or was it a therapeutically valid program for detoxification?

Although I was clearly on the mend, curiosity impelled me to try anything that could hasten the healing process. Accordingly, I rang the clinic in Los Angeles and spoke with the director, Michael Wisner.

"Do you think saunas could rid my body of its remaining chemicals and heavy metals?" I asked, after relating my history.

"Well, the program was tested on some people in Michigan," he said. "They were exposed to PBDEs[30] in 1973, when a mistake at the Michigan Chemical Corporation resulted in mixing large quantities of the flame retardant with a variety of cattle foods. Not only did the animals and livestock have to be destroyed, the contaminated meat and dairy products consumed during the nine months *before* the cause of the widespread illness was discovered left close to nine million people with measurable levels of PBDEs in their tissues and blood.[31]

"During a twenty-day sauna program," Wisner continued, "twenty-five percent of the toxins were found to have been removed, with corresponding improvement in reaction times and long-term memory."

A promising result, to be sure, but that left seventy-five percent of toxins still in the system and one couldn't take saunas forever. Even after fourteen months on the therapy, I was still shedding poisons that must have been in my body fat for years.

---

[30] Polybrominated diphenyl ethers, used as a flame retardant in plastics.

[31] As recently as November 2004, an Associated Press story reported that concentrations of PBDEs were found in the sediment of Lake Michigan, in supermarket foods, and in breast milk. "How the PBDEs and other chemicals get into Lake Michigan is still not clear," the story concluded.

Wisner also confirmed that Dr. Rae was building a sauna, modeled on the one in L.A., to replace the ECU. I told him about my test for chlorinated pesticides.

"I know the test," he said, "but it measures only the chemicals in the blood—it is the toxins in the body fat that matter." I agreed. "Anyway," he added, "before the program begins, we do tests to determine the level of these toxins."

It seemed worth exploring, so, as I was going to be in Los Angeles over Christmas visiting my daughters (my father had since died), I decided to do the program while there. I didn't expect saunas to be as effective as the juices, but thought they might be a useful adjunct.

I had been reading Carlos Castaneda's *The Teachings of Don Juan,* a literary success of the period that interested me because of the Don's apparent ability to sense energy lines without the use of a dowsing rod. His instruction to Castaneda to find his personal spot in which to sit, first by "feeling" it and then by "finding its color," suggested that in every culture, whether primitive or advanced, nature's way of identifying herself by color—even when the color is invisible—remains the same.

Concerning some of the Don's other teachings, however, I felt ambivalent. When one has experienced the malefic effect of chemicals on the brain as well as the body, the lure of mind-altering drugs as the door to perception seems a dangerous one. We need no "vastly complex system of beliefs" to experience exaltation—no mushroom, peyote, or jimson weed to become "a Man or Woman of Knowledge." Mescalito is all around us.

Reflecting on the way coming events cast their shadow before them, it occurred to me that food seemed to have been written into my destiny the day I entered my adoptive home. My father was a restaurateur whose catering career began in California, with low-priced dairy lunchrooms during the Depression. In the 1930s, he opened two newly popular drive-in restaurants, moved up-market in the 40s with two grill rooms in downtown Los Angeles, and ended his catering career in the 50s with the large restaurant concession at the Los Angeles airport.

My self-made father and I had little in common, apart from a mutual stubbornness and stiff-necked integrity. We clashed over almost everything, from dating to politics and from culture to capitalism. Yet what kept our estrangements from becoming permanent was an underlying respect for each other—and yes, love—a love that survived its greatest challenge during the Nixon-McCarthy era.

And now, I thought, here I am, as obsessed with food for the sake of survival as my father was for the sake of earning a living. I shuddered anew at the memory of that nerve-grating, knife-sharpening ritual that preceded his dismemberment of the Sunday roast; saw the two-inch steaks being delivered to our home by his wholesale supplier, and yearned anew (though less longingly now) for those rich desserts that crowned our Lucullan meals.

What would my father have thought had he known that forty years on, my health—perhaps even my life would depend on a diet the very opposite of the one on which I was being raised? Looking back, it seemed to me that I had been twice saved: first, by adoption into a loving home with indulgent parents who denied me nothing, and now, by a discipline of the most stringent self-denial—only this time, one that *I* had chosen to adopt.

CHAPTER THIRTY-FOUR

We do not inherit the land from our parents;
We hold the land in stewardship for our
grandchildren.

—Anon

My Christmas-at-a-clinic for 1986 was spent in a sauna, sweating out the old year and sweating in the new. I left London with the usual headache that began an hour into the flight. This one, however, was mild, so the journey was reasonably pleasant—as pleasant, that is, as any nine hours can be if spent in a metal box sharing germs with two hundred and fifty other people.

Michael Wisner had booked me into a motor hotel on Beverly Boulevard, chosen for its proximity to the clinic and its freedom from the sort of chemicals I would have been exposed to in a newly decorated, well-maintained hotel. The motel's maintenance was minimal and an excellent health food store two blocks away insured the seamless provision of organic vegetables and fruit.

I checked into HealthMed on the 15th of December for the preliminary tests, which included a complete medical examination, blood chemistries, toxicology screens, hair analysis for heavy metals, pulmonary function, electrocardiogram, urinalysis and a lengthy intelligence questionnaire. When I told the doctor I was doing the Gerson Therapy, she asked me to suspend the coffee enemas while I was there. I said I would try.

Two days later, the program began. Before entering the sauna, we were given a controlled dose of niacin (vitamin B_3) to trigger the release of toxins into the bloodstream. This was followed by a twenty-minute jog or brisk walk for the less fit.

"The jog acts with the niacin to increase the depth of circulation into your tissues," explained the supervisor, a beetle-browed fellow named Faxon, who took our blood pressure each morning and whose droll, laconic manner masked an ever-vigilant eye. "You must jog or walk in pairs and never sauna alone," he warned, "because you could have a flashback while unattended." A HealthMed flashback was a Gerson flare-up.

My jogging partners that morning were Sam—a balding ex-appliance salesman in his late sixties from Bakersfield— and Doris, a retired schoolteacher from Georgia, who, I was pleased to learn, was also staying at the motel. Choosing to walk briskly instead of jog, we exchanged our case histories along the way and discovered that we were chemical victims all three.

"I've been a heavy smoker since my teens," Sam confessed, "and I like to tinker in the garage on weekends—you know, with my car and doing a little woodwork—making things for the house. I thought I was a pretty healthy guy until a few years ago, when I developed emphysema and began to have a lot of other problems, so I guess the weed finally caught up with me."

Doris's story was similar to that of Louise, my housemate at Willie Mae's.

"One of the cleaners at school dumped a gallon of chlorine into the sink of the utility room next to my classroom," she said. "I had barely recovered from that when, without realizing it, the pilot light on my gas stove went out and I was exposed to carbon monoxide. A friend who worked in the office at school told me she got sick from the acetone that outgassed from the copier she used every day."

By the time I had skipped through my story our aerobic walk was over and we changed into our swimsuits (nudity was forbidden in the mixed sauna). Faxon recorded our starting weight and handed us each a clipboard, a form sheet, a sharpened pencil and two paper cups, containing salt and potassium tablets.

"You're to record the time each session begins and ends," he instructed, "along with the number of salt and potassium tablets you take, the glasses of water you drink, any symptoms that occur, and the total amount of sauna time completed each day. Heat exposure is from ten to thirty minutes, not more, followed by a ten- to fifteen-minute cooling-down period, with a cold shower and rest between each sauna. This is very important," he emphasized.

"The sauna room is ventilated and kept at about 140 degrees, unlike the usual 200 degrees maintained in health clubs. The lower temperature increases the excretion of toxins through the sweating mechanism without placing a strain on the heart. You'll be given daily supplements to replace the electrolytes, minerals, and vitamins lost during the sweating, with emphasis on calcium and magnesium, which you'll take as a drink."

The goal was five hours of sauna time per day, taken in half-hour segments. However, Faxon advised me to limit my first session to twenty minutes. I would have done so in any event, for by then I was feeling faintly ill. On quitting the sauna, he gave me a glass of the calcium-magnesium drink (Cal-Mag), which was a decided improvement over raw liver juice.

During the second session, my left ear began to pop and a strange odor emerged from my armpits. This was disconcerting, since I'd never had a problem with body odor. I confided my concern to Doris, who was in her second week of the program.

"I wouldn't worry," she said. "There was a girl here last week who gave off a strong body odor for two days. It must be the toxins coming out through your pores."

Later, when I queried Faxon about this, he confirmed it to be the case. "It's one of the detox signs we see in people who have taken street drugs," he said.

"But I've never taken street drugs."

"Well, it can also happen if you've had a lot of medicinal drugs, such as old antibiotics, anesthetics, tranquillizers, sleeping pills, painkillers—that sort of thing."

Why, then, I wondered, hadn't this symptom manifested before? Did saunas reach parts of the body the juices missed? More symptoms emerged during the second session and by the end of the third, Faxon decided I'd had enough for the first day. He weighed me again and gave me a large drink of unsaturated oils mixed with Keffir.

"The drink enhances fatty oil exchange and promotes fecal evacuation," he explained. "This is because only forty percent of toxins can be eliminated through the sweat glands."

In that case, I thought, why forbid enemas while provoking diarrhea?

On the walk back to the motel I felt thoroughly whacked. My head ached, my neck hurt, my ear kept popping and my left hip developed an arthritic twinge.

Altogether, a promising first day.

On the 19th, I woke at half-past five, feeling as though I had come down with the flu. The symptom cleared during the first sauna, but returned after the break, with more nausea and body odor. Again, Faxon restricted me to twenty-minute sessions.

I discovered that the employees were all Scientologists, although distinctly reticent about discussing the fact. No Hubbard books were on display, however, nor any pictures of Capt'n Ron looking jaunty in his yachting cap.

"The clinic's purpose is solely therapeutic," Faxon assured me, when I asked him about their absence. "It has nothing to do with drawing people into the religion." I saw no reason to doubt his statement during my four-weeks at HealthMed.

Two young women joined us in the sauna that morning—former patients in their twenties who were having one of the free maintenance sessions available to anyone who has completed the program. Bright and chatty, they told us about some of the symptoms they had witnessed during their detox sessions.

"When I was here a year ago," said the one in a blue swimsuit with brown hair and dark, intelligent eyes, "there was a middle-aged guy who'd been a heavy smoker. His legs began to ooze a brown liquid, as though nicotine was coming out of his pores. And I heard there was an LSD user who began tripping so badly in the sauna they made him stay in until he'd sweated it all out."

"What happened to me," said her bikini-clad friend, blonde hair pulled back in a ponytail, "was that my nose became all swollen and painful, and blue circles appeared under my eyes. I'd had a nose job two years before—and not only that, my body gave off an odor that smelled funny, like ethyl pentothal, which is the anesthetic they told me I was given at the time of my op."

I recalled Charlotte's story about the patient with the suture that worked its way out of her nose years after a rhinoplasty and wondered which chemicals were working their way out of my armpits? Chlorine? Dieldrin? Hexachlorobenzine?

Sam, bless his heart, was a bit of a drone—humming *Danny Boy* in the sauna and describing his symptoms in Proustian detail to anyone who would listen. Seeking a quieter ambiance, I decided to try the smaller sauna below, which Faxon told us we were not to use if alone. When I opened the door I found a young bloke there listening to a ball game on a transistor radio, so I returned to the sauna above. Better the drone I knew . . . .

On the 21st, I learned that a patient of Dr. Rae's had arrived from Texas. She appeared in the sauna the following day—a beautiful young woman, Lynn, who clearly had suffered a severe chemical assault, for her speech was slightly slurred and she moved with the same hesitancy I observed in the more seriously damaged victims.

Halfway through her first session she rose unsteadily and made her way out of the room. I assumed she had gone home, but when I entered the rest area for my break I found her there, drinking a glass of Cal-Mag. Curious to know her story, I introduced myself as a former patient of Dr. Rae's and asked if she would mind telling me what brought her to HealthMed.

"My husband and I built our million-dollar dream home in Dallas," she began, "but somehow the builder made a mistake. A pipe carrying trichloroethylene—that's a chemical used in dry cleaning—had been wrongly installed so that it emptied through a drain into my dressing room, which also served as an office for my decorating business. I spent hours there each day, inhaling the chemical without realizing it, and it attacked my nervous system.

"We're suing the builder, of course," she added, "but finances are running low. Meanwhile, my husband is also ill, and because the house is too contaminated to live in, our three young children are staying in a hotel back home with a helper."

My first thought was that Lynn should not be doing the program; she was much too ill.

"I hope you're not here alone," I said.

"My husband couldn't afford to come," she explained, "so I'm staying in a motel."

On confirming that we were staying at the same one, I invited her to join Doris and me when we walked to the clinic in the morning.

"Thank you," she said, "but I come later, you see, because I can't jog."

"Oh, of course. Well, then, perhaps on the walk back."

Faxon arrived just then to check on Lynn and wisely decided to send her home. I returned to the sauna and told Doris about our conversation.

"I'm concerned about Lynn walking to the clinic alone, Doris, especially when she starts to shed those chemicals in

232

earnest. Frankly, I'm not sure she should be doing the program."

"I suppose we could give her our room numbers in case she has an emergency at night," said Doris—"although," she added, her mind running on the same line as mine, "I don't know what we could do for her if she did."

Later that day, I shared my concern with Michael.

"What worries me, Michael, is that someone as ill as Lynn—especially if the chemicals are released too quickly into her bloodstream—could end up in a worse state than when she arrived. That's what happened to me when I left the ECU."

"Don't worry," he said, "we're keeping a close eye on her. In fact, we've scheduled some extra tests to determine whether she should stay in the program."

Walking back to the motel with Doris that afternoon, I noticed her pass her hand over her forehead several times.

"Are you all right, Doris?" I asked.

"It must be the perfume that girl was wearing in the changing room," she said. "It's brought back the headache I'd gotten rid of in the sauna."

"I know. It bothered me, too. I'm surprised they don't have a sign somewhere forbidding the use of scented products."

"I don't know how we can detoxify if we keep being exposed to the same chemicals that made us sick in the first place," grumbled Doris.

It was the litany of our lives, the lament of E.I. canaries everywhere as we topple from our perches, our toxic bodies a warning of the danger that lies ahead if we continue to pursue our mindless course. My heart ached for Doris, for I knew she would need more than saunas to repair the damage caused by that careless accident at school. I had suggested the Gerson Therapy, but she said she couldn't begin to afford it.

"I wonder why we're so heedless of our health, Doris," I mused—"I mean, as a nation, and so indifferent to the environmental problems we're creating for generations to come."

"Well," she sighed, "if we continue to procreate the way we're doing, there won't be any environment left for future generations to worry about."

"Of course, *that's* the fundamental problem, isn't it—and the most urgent, which no one has the courage to address for fear of treading on cultural or religious toes. NASA had better find a life-sustaining planet soon, for at the rate we're populating and polluting this one, we're going to need a cosmic bolt hole."[32]

"At least the Chinese have faced the problem by limiting families to one child," said Doris.

"Yes, but what if an only child dies? On the other hand, if we could send condoms to Africa and give women the means for controlling their fertility, think of the suffering they could be spared. I have only to see a picture of a starving child to know that not to be born is best!"

"Instead," said Doris, "we keep breeding and exploiting the earth as though its resources are inexhaustible."

"It's not even as though we need all the things that are creating the toxic waste being dumped into our oceans and landfills."

"No, but replacing them with non-toxic materials would cost a lot more."

"No more than the cost of cleaning up after a chemical spill. No more than the cost of our declining health and soaring medical bills. But who in Washington will defy the chemical and pharmaceutical lobbies, with their deep pockets and exorbitant bribes?"

"Well, let's hope *someone* in the government wakes up before it's too late," said Doris, without conviction.

---

[32] David Attenborough, the famous naturalist, recently observed: "There are three times as many people on earth as when I started making natural history programs 60 years ago . . . It seems to me there is a huge moral responsibility we have towards this planet." *The London Sunday Times,* September, 2008.

"Even if someone wakes up today," I said, "tomorrow is too late."

As long ago as 1984, Lee N. Davis wrote, in *The Corporate Alchemists:*

> Each year we are letting loose small quantities of new materials that do not occur naturally. Many have been specifically designed to be potent and toxic. Others become dangerous when overused, misused, or mixed with other substances. Such chemicals, borne by wind and water, have worked their way to the remotest portions of the globe and the farthest reaches of the atmosphere. We are literally surrounded by poisons. Their number increases annually. We have no idea what their ultimate effects will be.

Except that now, in the year 2010, we do.

CHAPTER THIRTY-FIVE

We are entering what may be called "the field
of vibrations," a field in which we may find
more wonders than the mind can conceive.
—Marconi

On December 22nd, I woke feeling headachy and vaguely ill. Something in the room was affecting me. It felt like an energy line, but I couldn't be sure because I had left my rod and color wheel in London. I was also inexpressibly tired, so I assumed I was having a flashback.

Although the doctor asked me to abjure coffee enemas, without their swift removal of the toxins released by the saunas, I'm not sure I would have stayed in the program. I did feel guilty about breaking the rules—though not so guilty I didn't break another one later that day when Sam broke into song and I fled again to the sauna below, this time finding it unoccupied.

We were joined in the changing room that morning by a pretty young college girl, Jennifer, who was fresh-faced and chubby, with light brown curls that fell in ringlets around her cheeks. She looked much too wholesome to be the drug-taking type (but then, what does the drug-taking type look like?), so, in my nosey way, I asked what brought her to HealthMed.

"I'm here to get NutraSweet out of my system," she said.[33]

---

[33] Trade name for aspartame, a chemical sweetener.

"NutraSweet?" I echoed, surprised.

"Yes, I've been trying to lose weight and was drinking lots of diet colas at college because I thought they were safe, but on the last day of school I passed out in my room. I don't know how long I lay there. When I regained consciousness almost everyone had gone and I found I was paralyzed. Fortunately, someone found me in time and the paralysis was only temporary, but it has affected my mind. By the time my doctor discovered the cause, some of the cells in my brain had been destroyed."

"But what makes him suspect NutraSweet?" I asked, more likely candidates springing to mind.

"Because the tests confirmed it," said Jennifer. "It's the aspartame. It's in all the sweeteners and diet colas. We found out that when aspartame is subjected to temperatures over 80 degrees it breaks down into methanol and methanol breakdown converts to formaldehyde, even in body heat."

"But if that's true, it should have been withdrawn years ago. Has your doctor reported this to the FDA?"

"Oh, yes," she said, "he has, but he doesn't think they'll do anything about it. He says the FDA protects the food and drug industries, not the public. Besides, Monsanto, who make aspartame, funds the American Diabetes Association [ADA], so the ADA exerts pressure on the FDA not to remove it. It's all about money."

Jennifer's experience was not the first to reveal the duplicity of government bureaucracies that were formed to protect the people, but protect the corporations instead. The problems with aspartame have been known to the FDA for years, yet Monsanto managed to have it incorporated into some 6,000 food products, such as diet sodas, yogurts, sugar-free desserts, candy, and chewing gum, in addition to those packets of sugar substitutes, like *Equal,* that sit so deceitfully on restaurant tables.

All about money, when it should be all about health.

In her book, *The Secret History of the War on Cancer,* Devra Davis cites a 1969 study of aspartame that was done with seven infant monkeys. "After a year of drinking milk flavored with the stuff," she writes, "one was dead and five had suffered severe epileptic seizures." A later study showed that "aspartame paired with the food flavoring monosodium glutamate produced brain tumors in rats." Manufacturers now hide MSG under a dozen different names, such as "hydrolyzed soy protein," etc. It is in far more foods than we realize.

On the 27th of December, the soles of my feet began to ache while I was in the sauna. A strong odor was also issuing again from my pores. Lynn, however, was showing a marked improvement that day. Her speech was fluent and she was steadier on her feet. She rarely stayed for the last sauna, so Doris and I invited her to walk with us back to the motel.

To avoid the traffic fumes on Beverly Boulevard, we went through a back alley that led past a row of garages belonging to the apartment buildings that faced the street. One of the garage doors ahead was open and as we approached it, Lynn suddenly gasped, "Oh, no!" and her legs began to buckle. We caught her in time, but didn't know what happened until we drew abreast of the garage. Then Doris and I, too, caught the whiff of motor oil. We managed to get Lynn safely to the motel, but all the progress she made in the sauna that day was undone in a matter of seconds.

In her room, Lynn collapsed on the bed and lay motionless with her eyes closed.

"Is there anything we can do for you, Lynn?" we asked, knowing there wasn't, for she was in that realm of suffering beyond human comforting or help. Two small frown lines appeared between her brows before she managed to say, in a barely audible voice,

"I need to eat some greens, but I don't have any. Anyway, I don't think I have the strength to cook."

"You don't have to," I said. "I was going to make a salad for dinner, so I'll make enough for two."

While Doris stayed with Lynn, I went downstairs and threw some greens together with a tomato, a hard-boiled egg, slices of cucumber, and a yogurt and chive dressing. Adding some fruit to the tray, I returned to Lynn's room and placed the tray on her nightstand.

"I'll be going to the health food store tomorrow, Lynn," I said. "If there's anything you need I can shop for you at the same time."

Doris helped Lynn raise herself into a sitting position while I made a mental note of the few items she requested. There being nothing more we could do for her we returned to our rooms, for Doris and I, too, had begun to react to the motor oil.

Too tired to make another salad, I opened a tin of salmon, which I ate without appetite, and went to bed. I wanted to sleep, but thoughts of Lynn kept me awake. What further damage had that brief exposure done to her immune system? How could a glass of Keffir and oils clear from her body all the toxins being released into her bloodstream? I dreaded to think how *I* might have fared had my first choice been saunas instead of Gerson.

At the grocery store the next day, I added some flaxseed oil and bottles of carrot juice to Lynn's shopping list. There couldn't have been a live enzyme left in the juice, but it was better than nothing. When I reached Lynn's room, she was still desperately ill.

"I don't know when I'll be able to do the saunas again," she said, in a small voice flat with fatigue.

"Well, if I were you, I shouldn't try," I said, "until you've had a talk with Michael about your condition."

That night, I had trouble sleeping again. My throat was dry and I felt a headache coming on. Some time before midnight my feet began to quiver, as if a tiny motor had been embedded in each foot. I remembered feeling a similar sort of vibration that last night at the clinic. Could an earthquake be imminent? I had read somewhere that those who experience symptoms before a quake do so because of magnetite in the brain, which acts as a seismic sentry—or perhaps it was seismic sensor. If there should be an earthquake, I reflected, what do I do? Stand in a doorway? Shelter under a table?

The next morning, I turned on the radio for the news and heard that a mild earthquake had occurred in the Hayward district of the Bay City area at 7:28 a.m.—3.5 on the Richter scale.

I had no idea where the Hayward district was, but later I learned it was about 300 miles north of Los Angeles. Surely that was too distant for premonitory vibrations to be felt in Beverly Hills. Still, the distance between Mexico City and La Gloria was five times greater—although the quake was five times stronger, too. If my symptoms the night before *were* due to the coming quake, were they weaker this time because the quake was weaker or because my immune system was stronger?

The thought that I might be subject to these energies for the rest of my life was so disheartening, I shoved it away. Hoping it was just coincidence, I recorded the incident in my diary and turned my attention to the more pressing matter of breakfast.

Meanwhile, without intending to, I seemed to be giving Faxon a hard time. When I told him on the 30th that I had taken an enema the night before to relieve a headache, he looked faintly aggrieved. When I admitted to having had one the night before that, he sucked at his teeth and scowled. I had already blotted my copybook by suggesting that coffee enemas be added to the program. I did feel the teeniest bit guilty about confessing to only two, but, as Heinrich Heine said, "God will forgive me; c'est son metier."

Doris was ill that day and staying in her room. Sam had finished the program and decamped the day before, so I was assigned a new jogging partner—a lady of a certain age, Mitzi, who was blondish, fiftyish and trim of figure, with a gamine haircut and pixie-cute personality. Relieved to be spared Sam's lugubrious narratives, I welcomed this new companion, for she promised to be an invigorating change. Mitzi was more than invigorating—she was one of life's chatterboxes.

"I think I should warn you that I'm kind of hyper," she began, as we set out on our walk. "I mean, I'm so hyper that one of my colleagues at work said to me, 'Mitzi,' she said, 'they could bury you under a concrete slab and you'd come right back up like a weed, even if you had to crack open the concrete!' Tee hee! They all think I'm a card at the office."

Extruding verbiage like ectoplasm, Mitzi, who worked in a department store, had the kind of chirpiness that forestalls any need for response on the part of the listener. We had scarcely begun our power walk when she cried, "Wait!" I stopped, while Mitzi reached into her pocket and withdrew a chocolate bar.

"I shouldn't be eating this, you know," she said, unwrapping it with a greedy giggle. "My doctor read me the riot act when I told him I was coming here to get rid of the chemicals in my system. 'Mitzi,' he said, 'I think you're crazy. Your trouble is allergy, allergy! And chocolate is the worst thing for you, you've got to give it up!' But I can't," she whimpered, making a moue. "I mean—it's so *addictive*! I would *kill* for chocolate—it's more addictive than sex! Here—want a bite?"

As a recovering chocoholic in my sixteenth month of abstinence, I did not welcome Mitzi's generosity. *There but for the grace of Gerson,* thought I, keeping a grip on my self-control. To her credit, Mitzi had a healthy sense of humor about herself, although she managed to get up the noses of several people—Faxon's in particular, whose laid-back feathers she kept ruffling by calling him "Fraxon."

"By the way," said Mitzi, as we set out on our walk two days later, "what star sign were you born under?"

"Scorpio. Why?"

"Why, I'm Scorpio, too! How *amazing!* Do you know what your rising sign is?"

"Yes. Cancer."

"I have Gemini rising. No wonder we get on so well. I told Fraxon you're the only person I like to walk with because you walk fast, like me, and are so interesting to talk to. I'm an amateur astrologer, you know, and a very old soul.

Oh, it's all there in my chart. You won't believe this, but once, in a former life . . . ."

And so, interminably, on.

That afternoon, Lynn appeared in the sauna, her mental confusion suggesting someone in the early stages of Alzheimer's. I suspected chemicals played a role in that condition as well and was glad when Faxon sent her home early, although concerned about her making it safely to the motel on her own.

Plodding home on the last day of the year with low spirits, a raw throat and a pounding head, I missed Doris's level-headed company. She was still ill, but had finished the program and would be going home the next day. If only I knew some affordable way in which she could be helped.

Lying in bed that night as midnight approached, and unable to sleep, I thought of my daughters who were welcoming the New Year with Amy's birth-father and his family. I would have been with them, but he lived some distance away and I didn't want to drive home in the early morning hours. Instead, I reflected, here I am, spending New Year's Eve in a run-down motel, when I should be in London greeting the coming year with a few close friends and subdued expectations.

Around 2:30 a.m., I woke to feel the familiar quivering in my feet. I tried to ignore it, but it was annoying enough to keep me awake for over an hour.

The next morning, I switched on the radio:

> There has been a mild earthquake in Palm Springs, about 120 miles from Los Angeles, 3.6 on the Richter scale.

CHAPTER THIRTY-SIX

All are but parts of one stupendous whole,
whose body nature is, and God the soul.
—Alexander Pope

"Oh, yes," said Mitzi, as we pretended to power walk around the block on the third day of the New Year. "I've been through all that new-age stuff—tarot, channeling, OBEs.[34] Once, when I was out of my body, I had the most *amazing* experience! I was traveling in a little spaceship all by myself, faster than the speed of light, when these *amazing* beings appeared! I knew they were cosmic beings, not aliens, because they had no faces and were from a much more advanced civilization. Anyway, while they were showing me my former lives, they took me to the planet Sirius and they said to me, 'Mitzi,' they said, 'you won't remember this, but many lifetimes ago, you were a high priestess here on this planet.'"

"Oh, do tell me—what is Sirius like?"

"Well, it's not like earth at all. The buildings are all round and made of glass and you can walk right through the walls, only of course your feet don't touch the ground. Only very old souls reincarnate on Sirius—those who have evolved over many lifetimes."

Mitzi was still on her cosmic canter in the sauna, when I thought I felt a slight tremor in the bench on which we were sitting. I wanted to ask if she felt it, too, but Mitzi was in

---

[34] Out-of-body experiences.

mid-flow and by the time she drew breath, the tremor had stopped. Later that day, a second earthquake occurred near Palm Springs, also measuring 3.6 on the Richter scale.

Intrigued by these synchronicities, I consulted my diary that evening to see if a time pattern emerged between the onset of certain symptoms and the arrival of a quake. Depending upon the strength of the temblor and its distance from Los Angeles, there seemed to be an interval of from four to six hours between the two. I hadn't noted the time of the tremor that morning, nor of the quake that afternoon, but if the former occurred around 10:30 a.m. and the latter between two and four in the afternoon, the interval would have fallen within that range.

All the same, three coincidences did not make a premonition.

That same day, we learned that Lynn had dropped out of the program and was undergoing some neurological tests before they would let her continue.

"Her condition has deteriorated rapidly," Faxon told us.

My heart dropped into my stomach. If only we hadn't taken that fatal path through the alley.

On the 4th of January, two newcomers appeared in the sauna—young married women who were trying to get old LSD out of their systems before becoming pregnant.

"Yeah, we used to do drugs," said one, "but now that we want to have kids, we thought we'd better get clean first."

While talking with them, it occurred to me that we hadn't been given any dietary advice to go with our other instructions. I asked Michael Wisner about this later that day.

"We don't believe in imposing an additional burden on people while they're doing the program," he explained.

Burden? Different therapy, different approach: nutrition as burden instead of builder.

On the 5th of January, I woke at half-past midnight with my body gently vibrating and my feet thrumming as though hooked up to that generator again. The symptoms were stronger this time, so I recorded them in my diary in case another seismic surprise was on its way.

Waking a few hours later, I switched on the radio and heard that an earthquake had occurred off the Aleutian Islands—6.4 on the Richter scale.

Now, it is one thing to sense the vibrations of a coming quake when they are under one's feet, so to speak, but quite another to imagine they could be felt when occurring off a distant shore. Having experienced a number of so-called paranormal events, I was accustomed to taking the inexplicable in my stride, but to imagine the least connection between my thrumming feet in Beverly Hills and shifting subterranean plates in the Aleutian Islands, strained even my credulity.

Still, if the human nervous system can be affected by a fractured earth energy line or the emanation from a polluted stream, why shouldn't it sense an impending displacement of the earth itself? After all, earth, sea, and air are all part of one planetary whole, with which we are in constant, if not always conscious communion.

I still had no answer for why my symptoms were stronger before the more distant quake than before the nearer and weaker one in Palm Springs. Could it be that the vibrations in the Aleutians traveled along the ocean floor— their power increasing, like a tsunami, in inverse ratio to their distance from the quake's epicenter?[35] I resolved to consult Tributsch's book when I got home, to see if there were any relevant clues I might have missed on first reading.

Reflecting on the subtle power of water, I recalled something I had read by Giorgio Piccardi, who was Director of the Institute of Physical Chemistry in Florence, Italy, at the time:

---

[35] Tributsch writes that as tsunamis race across the ocean, they pound the rock formations beneath the sea floor, and because sound travels faster through rock than water, animals have time to flee.

> Water is sensitive to extremely delicate influences and is capable of adapting itself to the most varying circumstances to a degree attained by no other liquid. Perhaps it is even by means of water and the aqueous system that the external forces are able to react on living organisms.

For as long as I could remember water had been my native element. Much of my childhood was spent at the bottom of a swimming pool, searching for pennies my brother and I had thrown in—or, with scarves attached to my swimsuit, pretending to be a sinuous Ondine, twisting and turning in the silent depths to watch the silken squares make graceful arabesques in my wake.

Even my astrological chart was awash with watery signs, including a "grand trine" in water, whatever that meant, though I felt sure Mitzi could tell me. It was my love of rain that made the English climate so congenial to my spirit and me so peculiar to my English friends. And it was a narrow stream running under my bed that led to the discovery of my body's response to its radiations.

We were in the sauna that afternoon when Faxon opened the door to tell us that Lynn may have suffered some brain damage and had dropped out of the program.

"Her brother has arrived from Texas to take her home," he added. "She's downstairs now, if you want to say good-bye to her."

The shock of seeing Lynn in a wheelchair—so beautiful and so broken—was heartrending. As we each bent down to kiss her good-bye, her eyes filled with tears. We managed to withhold ours until she had gone, but as her brother wheeled her toward the door I slipped a hastily scribbled note into his pocket, urging them to look into the Gerson Therapy. I knew they wouldn't. Why should they, when the alternative options they had already tried—too late—had failed?

"Lynn's blood tests showed an exceptionally high level of trichloroethylene in her body," Faxon told us later, "a thousand times higher than it should have been. It was this chemical, which is employed mainly in the dry-cleaning process, that she had been breathing for months as it came up through a pipe into her dressing room."

On the evening of January 8th—a Thursday—I was fixing supper in my room, when I thought I felt a faint tremor in my lower legs. It was so weak that, were it not for my habit of hyper-vigilance, I might not have noticed it. For a moment I considered lying down, for symptoms were always more pronounced when I was prone, but the vibration was so mild and I was so hungry, I decided to eat instead. Once in bed, however, the tremor was unmistakable.

Some time after midnight I woke and was unable to go back to sleep, so I turned on the bedside radio. At half-past twelve, the news bulletin reported that an earthquake had occurred off the coast of Japan—"On Friday afternoon, measuring 6.9 on the Richter scale."

To imagine the remotest connection between an off-shore quake in Japan and my symptom of the night before suggests serious lunacy. Moreover, I had no idea what the time difference was between California and Japan. Nonetheless, I recorded the details in my diary and went back to sleep.

(On the 5th of July, 1989, while transcribing the Health-Med chapter in London, I came upon the above incident in my diary, which I had forgotten. I decided to ring the Information Bureau of the *Daily Telegraph* to ascertain the distance, as well as the difference in time zones between Tokyo and Los Angeles. Japan, they informed me, is 16 hours ahead of Los Angeles and the distance is roughly 5,450 miles.)

I hadn't bothered to note the time of the tremor, but I usually ate around seven, which would have been roughly noon in Japan on the following day. The quake occurred on Friday afternoon, and was reported at 5:30 p.m. their time. My grasp of numbers is shaky at best, but if it happened within the preceding hour—say, around 4:30 p.m., this would have placed my symptom—if that is what it was—a few hours before the quake.

This was the last such anomaly to occur during my four-week stay in Los Angeles. That these synchronicities happened only when I was on the Mexican-California littoral confirmed their purely telluric origin. There was nothing remotely psychic about the sensings. My peculiar body had simply reacted like a pendulum to a subtle disturbance in the earth—the way a dowser's rod reacts to an underground stream, pure or polluted, that flows beneath his feet.

I am persuaded that far more people than are aware of it experience some sort of physical change, however slight, hours or even days before an earthquake, assuming they are within its radius—and, in some cases, even if they are not. If they fail to notice the change or make the connection, it is because they haven't acquired the habit of listening to their body and monitoring its symptoms.

The awareness is all.

My last day at HealthMed, I met with the doctor for a final checkup and review of my various tests. As anticipated, they showed a significant reduction in the remaining chemicals in my system.

"The real test, though," I told Michael, as we said good-bye, "will be if I can reach Heathrow without having a headache on the plane."

Happily, the flight home was headache-free, though whether because of the saunas or a strengthened immune system, I'm not sure. I believe both contributed to this welcome liberation. I did feel saunas could be a worthy adjunct to the Gerson therapy in the growing problem of environmental illness. However, I would discourage anyone with a severely damaged immune system from choosing them as a first resort. Had I begun with saunas instead of Gerson, I might have ended up the way Lynn did—the way Doris wrote that she did, too, in a letter I received from her two weeks after my return to London.

"I've been going downhill ever since I returned home," it read. "Maybe I should have stayed longer, the way that LSD user was forced to stay in the sauna until he was completely clear. I don't know what I'll do now.

"By the way," she added, "I understand that shortly after you left, Mitzi dropped out of the program and returned home in high dudgeon. Some altercation with Faxon, I believe."

CHAPTER THIRTY-SEVEN

To the observers of nature without name, title
or career for their contributions to the
progress of Science.
—Helmut Tributsch[36]

My first act on returning home was to read through the
Snakes book again for any passages that could throw light
on the synchronicities that occurred in Los Angeles. A
possible clue appeared in the chapter on the piezoelectric
effect:

> If electrostatic charges do move from the
> ground into the atmosphere, and if their lib-
> eration and neutralization produces long elec-
> tromagnetic waves and changes in the electric
> field, then sensitive people must feel the ap-
> proach of an earthquake.

Searching through other books in my library, I found this
passage in Lyall Watson's *Neophilia:*

> We know now that earthquakes make our
> whole planet ring like a gong, setting up long
> wave, low-frequency oscillations that go on
> for an hour or more and can be measured
> anywhere on earth. These vibrations occur at
> frequencies from seven to fourteen cycles per

---

[36] Dedication, *When the Snakes Awake.*

second, and the fascinating thing about them is that they not only accompany, but also precede the actual occurrence of a quake.

And in *Supernature,* Watson observes:

> It has now been discovered that an earthquake is also accompanied by, and preceded by, periods of low-frequency vibrations that fall into the range from seven to fourteen cycles per second. These start minutes before the first obvious shocks of the quake itself and provide an early-warning system to which many species seem to respond.
> … Some people, particularly women and children, are also sensitive to these frequencies. The fact that the frequencies coincide with those that make people disturbed and ill would account for the wild, unreasoning fear that goes with an earthquake.

"Wild, unreasoning fear" was what I experienced that night at La Gloria, when the only cause I could find for my physical distress was an environment that had gone haywire. If my symptoms in Los Angeles lacked the element of fear, it may have been because the quakes were weaker, or because those in the Aleutians and Japan were farther away. Or—as seems to me more likely—because fifteen months of the therapy had restored my immune system to the point where I was no longer as sensitive as before to geopathic stress.

Further evidence of progress was the return of a kind of energy I had almost forgotten I once possessed. Flare-ups were few and milder when they came, but as I still had toxins to shed, I decided to hasten the process by adding a weekly sauna to the regime.

Accordingly, I joined a nearby health club, whose equipment I couldn't use because of the disinfectant in the workout room and in whose pool I couldn't swim because of the chlorine. In the sauna my nose recoiled from the many perfumed lotions the women employed. One woman kept rubbing her body with an oil so fragrant it forced me to flee—and to abandon the health club altogether.

Eventually, I found a less salubrious establishment where, if I arrived when it opened in the morning, I usually had the sauna to myself. By June 1987, I was having two saunas a week with detox symptoms similar to, though not as strong as, those I experienced at HealthMed.

A final flare-up of mindless anger occurred on the 28th, but this time it lasted only a day—and this time I didn't need to bash a pillow.

Bronya, meanwhile, having enjoyed a month's vacation during my absence, was as disputatious as ever when I returned. Resigned though I was to her labyrinthine work methods, her need to score points was beginning to get up my nose.

In February, for instance, I remarked that I was only a month away from achieving the therapy's eighteen-month milestone for cancer.

"Isn't it ironic, Bronya," I observed, "that with a father in the restaurant business, for whom meat was the focus of every meal, my health is being restored by a vegetarian regime the very opposite of the one on which I was raised?"

"How do you know it's not just the placebo effect?" she challenged. "Maybe the therapy only works because you want it to."

"If that were so," I replied, with a twitch of irritation, "why did none of the other therapies I tried work as well? God knows, I wanted them to."

"But it's all in your *mind,* I tell you," she cried, with an intensity quite out of proportion to the subject at hand. "The therapy only works because you *believe* that it will!"

Too weary to wonder how a simple statement of fact had become a psychological issue, I said, "In that case, Bronya, why did I choose the hardest therapy of all to believe in?" But she just gave me one of her pitying little smiles, which I knew meant, "Don't blind me with logic, I've won the debate and the subject is closed."

My patience with this sort of thing had been growing thin and on the 5th of April it finally cracked. Bronya was dispatched, taking with her on the day of departure—in addition to her suitcase—so many plastic bags containing heaven knew what, they filled the back of the taxi I hired in which to send her home.

Clive came to town on the 23rd for a meeting of the Dowsing Society, arriving early to show me some of his latest discoveries before we left for the hall. I was still keenly involved in his research, only now more as an observer than a participant. And now that I no longer needed his help (or no longer believed that I did), our relationship was more relaxed— even quite playful at times.

We had already discussed the earthquake incidents on my return from L.A., at which time Clive declared himself convinced my symptoms were premonitory. He reaffirmed this that afternoon.

"Then you're quite sure it wasn't just coincidence?" I asked, testing his certainty.

"Oh, there's no doubt in my mind you were picking up the vibrations," he said, entwining his fingers across his chest in the familiar gesture. Few things took Clive by surprise or struck him as beyond the realm of the possible.

"Even the quakes off the Aleutians and Japan?" I goaded, testing us both.

"Of course. Given your sensitivity to earth energies, I suspect you're tuned in to some sort of earthquake frequency. You're like a spider on a web, aren't you? Even the smallest tug at the farthest extremity of the web can still be sensed by the spider."

Not the happiest simile for an arachnophobe, but I knew what he meant. Our dowsing experiments had proved again and again the irrelevance of distance and the interconnected-ness of all things. I was going to miss those experiments— the failures, especially—for, paradoxically, it was often the failures that proved the reality of those invisible forces that fill what we so mistakenly think of as empty space.

Bronya was replaced by a forty-three-year-old American hippie, Devla, who said she was familiar with the Norwalk machine because she had worked for a year making juices at a holistic retreat. When she added that she, too, was a vegetarian, I engaged her on the spot; at least we would be as one on the subject of nutrition.

It soon became clear, however, that what Devla *hoped* she would be doing, apart from making juices, was holding someone's hand and being "spiritual." Preparing a meal, picking up food that fell on the floor—even making the juices—was not really her thing. As slow as Bronya and arguably more disorganized, each time she ran the Norwalk machine (a procedure I thought she knew), she referred to a piece of paper on which she had written the instructions.

After four testing months, I had to tell Devla that, sadly, it was not going to work. She took it in good part, the way she took all life's vicissitudes—a quality I greatly admire and would have cherished, had it been accompanied by a modicum of efficiency.

On the eve of her departure, Devla poked her head around the door and said, ever so winsomely, "Before I go, I just wanted you to know that my special gift is to comfort and heal. I thought I would leave that with you."

"Thank you, Devla," I said, "I appreciate your sharing that with me."

What I wanted to say was, "Your special gift may be dancing with moonbeams, but my special need is for someone to chop wood, carry water."

By August 1987, I had progressed to the modified regime, which meant fewer juices and, happily, no further need for someone to live in. Devla was replaced in turn with three foreign students who were in London to improve their English and who came for a few hours a day to make two juices and prepare a meal.

First there was Heiki—half German, half-Spanish and my favorite. Then came Anna—Italian, fair-haired and studious, with whom I refreshed my once-fluent Italian. Last, came the Portuguese Fatima, who was dark, diligent, and prim. All three were so engaging in their different ways, and so delightful to have around, that when the time came for each to return home, a bit of my heart went with her. But they had better things to do with their young lives than grind vegetables for a dotty ex-pat American.

Although even a mild flare-up was now rare, several long-standing conditions proved resistant to the therapy's overall success. The hay fever was genetic, of course—inherited from my birth mother, which I learned when I met her in 1974. As for my few remaining problems, I hoped Jung was wrong when he wrote, "The meaning and purpose of a problem seem to lie not in its solution, but in our working at it incessantly."

In October, I experienced a final bout of discouragement—with writing, with myself and with the therapy, which was consuming most of my time now that I was doing the kitchen chores. It was hard not to feel that Someone Up There didn't want the book on adoption to be finished.

On the 27th, I moaned to my diary:

> Have never felt so discouraged. I work without feedback, plodding on, year after year, like poor old Sisyphus, without ever reaching the end. Montaigne wrote that he suffered from "the disease of writing books and being ashamed of them when they are finished." But his were finished. I just have the disease.

By December, however, the picture looked brighter. I was no longer waking with stiffness in my limbs, sickness in my body or depression in my soul. When I worked, it was as though a blanket of cotton wool had been removed from my brain, enabling me to unsnarl some of the mangled syntax that appeared so distressingly on every page.

As for my physical energy, it could scarcely be contained. On the 5th, I donned a track suit and jogged up the Fulham road to the new Conran store, marveling (on the slower walk back) at the distance I had covered.

That evening, I watched a television program titled, *The Sixth Sense,* about the ability of animals to sense things of which humans are unaware.

"Scorpions in particular," said the narrator (referring to the crustaceous kind), "are sensitive to air currents and are endowed with almost mystical powers for foretelling earthquakes and volcanic eruptions . . . Water animals," he added, "sense vibrations of a different nature."

Noting that water is a known conductor of energy, Tributsch observes, "Fish and aquatic animals seem to suffer more intensely from the consequences of earthquakes than do land animals."

Perhaps, then, I really was that "queer fish" Clive so often accused me of being—not always in jest.

Five days before Christmas 1987, I flew, headache-free, to Los Angeles to spend the holiday with my daughters, staying this time with my favorite cousin, Arlene. I had stayed with her before, enduring the perfumed scents in her guest room as the price I had to pay for the fun of her company. The scents were still there, but now I was able to tolerate them, if only just.

I also fell spectacularly off my diet, for temptation lurked in every corner of my cousin's kitchen: in the candy-filled dish on the counter, the pastries in the refrigerator, and the cartons of ice cream that stood cheek by jowl with packages of meat in the freezer.

Arlene and her husband, Larry, followed the usual American diet of meat, fish, carbohydrates, lashings of butter, salt on everything and rich desserts at the end. Larry, a doctor, drank diet colas to keep his weight down. Years later, when he died of Alzheimer's, I wondered if the aspartame in the colas had contributed to the disease. With the exception of meat I ate everything on offer, telling myself that I had been good for so long and was doing so well, I deserved a proper binge.

On the afternoon of January 2nd, 1988, I felt unusually tired and went to bed early with a mild headache. Shortly after midnight, I woke with a parched throat and the familiar tingling in my feet. This time, however, my hands were flaring too, and as that was my classic food allergy symptom, I assumed I was reacting to all the forbidden foods I had been eating.

The next morning, I turned on the radio as usual for the news:

> There has been a small earthquake six miles southeast of Pasadena at 3:52 this morning. Its magnitude was 3.2 on the Richter scale.

Only a baby quake, then, and Pasadena was not that far away.

At dinner that evening, my feet began to thrum gently under the table. Toward midnight, I woke again with a headache. The following day, an aftershock of the Pasadena quake occurred in Orange County, around 3:00 p.m., 3.6 on the Richter scale.

These were the only earthquakes to occur during that visit home. If I add them to those of the year before, the number of symptoms that may—or may not—have been premonitory, were six.

At the end of 1989, after living twenty of the most rewarding, if challenging years of my life in England, I returned to California to be near my daughters and settled in Santa Barbara. When the Northridge earthquake struck on January 17, 1994—at 6.7 the worst quake in the Los Angeles basin since 1971—the only anomaly I recorded in my diary the day before was a feeling of mild illness.

With this proof that I was no longer that spider on a web, trembling at the slightest tug from the farthest extremity, I knew my immune system had been restored—as much as it could be, that is, given the ongoing exposures to pollution that no one can escape.

At long last—and oh, so thankfully—I was again a normal human being.

CHAPTER THIRTY-EIGHT

The most formidable barrier to the advancement of Science is the conventional wisdom of the prevailing group.
—C.H. Waddington

In 1997 I moved to North Carolina and in September of 2004, I needed another operation on my toes. They had not healed properly after the surgery in London, due to my inability to tolerate the pins. Now, however, nineteen years had passed; I had a restored immune system and perhaps I was no longer as sensitive to the metal as before.

The new surgeon could not have been more genial, or less like his odious predecessor. Sandy-haired and smiling, Dr. Hauser examined my toes and explained that in order to correct the problem, he would need to put a pin in each toe. I expressed concern and told him of my previous experience.

Instead of the slightly scoffing response I expected, he handed me a leaflet, saying, "This will explain some of the postoperative reactions you might have." I opened the leaflet and the first words I saw were, *"You may have an allergic reaction to the steel pins or the nylon sutures."*

Well, well, I thought, podiatry has come a long way since 1985—at least on this side of the pond. No doubt observant foot surgeons were finally compelled to acknowledge what was under their noses, quite literally, for years.

Delighted to have found a doctor who was both sympathetic and informed, and encouraged by my strengthened immune system, I decided to risk the pins. I did feel some apprehension about postoperative pain—the memory of that night in the hospital having burned itself into my cortex.

On the morning of the operation, I declined the nurse's offer of a pre-op Valium, "to calm your nerves," since I had no nerves that needed calming. When I came to in the recovery room, the first words I heard were, "Would you like something to drink? A Coke? Ginger ale, or water? Or something to eat? Graham crackers or saltines?" Nothing could have mattered less at that moment than food, but I accepted the water, having prepared a bowl of oatmeal and fruit for when I returned home.

Now that my toes were pinned I had no need of a cast, only a funny-looking shoe and the help of a walker for the first few days. To my surprise, I required only one painkiller after the operation. In fact, the whole experience would have been problem-free, had it not been for my own stupidity the following day. Due to an unusual number of visitors, I was on my feet with the walker for much of the time, when I should have stayed in bed with my foot raised, as the surgeon instructed.

First came the gardener, seeking advice about where to plant a cherry tree, followed by the heating engineer, to see about a problem with the thermostat. Then a member of my writing group arrived to collect my critique of her story for the meeting that night, which I could not attend. Lastly, a friend came to help me prepare some documents to put in my safe deposit box at the bank. This could have waited for weeks—but, as I discovered only later, my friend's sense of urgency was due to the fact that one of the documents was my will, in which, as she knew, she was the main beneficiary.

Instead of staying in bed as I should have done, I was on my feet searching for papers in a file cabinet and sitting with her on the sofa, going through the documents. It did strike me as odd that she seemed scarcely to notice my condition—but then, I didn't realize her concern lay elsewhere.

If my willingness to be up and about the day after surgery implied that it was fine to be on my feet, I had only myself to blame. When one is blessed with unusual energy in one's seventies, the need to remain in bed for any purpose other than sleep is intolerable. As a result of this infraction, my toes bled profusely for the next few days—and the friend is no longer in my life.

When Dr. Hauser rang that evening to see how I was getting on, I had to admit that I had been up a bit that day.

"You mean you haven't been staying in bed with your foot raised?"

"No," I confessed, ashamed to reveal how foolish I'd been. "And my toes are bleeding quite a lot, but I suppose that's normal."

"No, it is not," he said, sharply. "That will increase the swelling. You should have been in bed with an ice pack on your foot." He might also have added that now I would need more than one painkiller a day.

On the 27th, I saw Dr. Hauser to have my blood-soaked dressing changed.

"Because of the excessive bleeding," he said, "I'm going to have to put you on antibiotics for ten days to prevent infection."

"Oh no!" I wailed, *"More* antibiotics—when I've just spent two years getting rid of the old ones!"

On the 6th of October, Dr. Hauser removed the stitches in my toes—so gently I scarcely felt a thing.

"You seem to be tolerating the pins quite well," he observed, examining my foot before applying the new dressing.

The contrast between this experience and the one nineteen years earlier was so marked that, had it not been for a sense of propriety and the fear of alarming him, I would have leapt from the table and given Dr. Hauser a hug.

By the 12th, however, I could feel a mild pressure building up in my toes. Suspecting the pins, I realized that although my body had tolerated them for four weeks, it could not have done so indefinitely.

"I can see you're reacting to the pins," said the surgeon, when we met two days later, "because there's a bit more swelling here than there should be."

He began to remove them—a *very* painful process this time, although it was not his fault; I have an absurdly low threshold of pain. Within moments of their removal, the relief was palpable. By the time I was heading home in the car, my toes felt as though they had bathed in a cool, soothing stream.

This proof that my body still could not harbor a foreign substance for long, suggested that once an immune system has been severely compromised, complete recovery may not be possible. Whether the human body was designed to cope with the many man-made substances it can no longer avoid, I will leave for future generations to decide. That I tolerated the stainless steel for as long as I did was proof of a healing I would not have thought possible ten years earlier.

Some weeks later, during a follow-up visit, I was discussing this evidence of a vestigial sensitivity with Dr. Hauser, when he told me of an experience he had with an equally sensitive patient whose foot he had operated on.

"When her leg began to swell inside the cast two months after the operation, I decided to remove the screw. Even before it was completely out, she said, 'Oh, that feels much better!' Another patient reacted to the soluble sutures, which kept rising to the surface of her skin. I would cut off the bit that stuck out, only to have the rest of the suture slowly emerge and have to be cut off as well. "

Shades of Charlotte's rhinoplasty patient again.

"So you see," he added, with an engaging grin, "you're not the only patient whose body has tried to reject a foreign object."

Oh! I thought—if only I had heard those words nineteen years earlier, what suffering they could have spared me!

Three weeks later, I saw Dr. Hauser for a final checkup. He was examining my toes, when, to his surprise, he discovered he had overlooked a suture in one toe.

Had he not told me it was there, I would not have known.

CHAPTER THIRTY-NINE

It is no measure of health to be well-adjusted
to a profoundly sick society.
—Krishnamurti

When I began this account of my search for health some years ago, I hoped it might end with all my questions answered and most of my physical problems healed. Life, however, is not so obliging. Although I now have a restored immune system and geopathic stress is a distant nightmare, perfect health remains a work in progress, with a few more revisions still to come.

I also hoped to find an easier method of detoxification than Gerson's for those who found his regime too difficult to follow—and even for those of us who didn't. After all, no one approach works for everyone, whether it be alternative or allopathic, and in certain cases genetic predisposition limits the curative options.

Gerson's genius, however, was not that he found a cure for cancer, but that he found a nutritional therapy that restores the body's immune system, thus enabling it to correct whatever is out of balance—be it cancer, lupus, or a migraine headache.

When Hippocrates wrote, "Let food be your medicine, let medicine be your food," he was not referring to the denatured, tarted-up and processed artifact that we call "food" today. Overfed and undernourished, we have surrendered our well-being to the food merchants, whose lure of "convenience" means whatever is most convenient (and profitable) for them, not what is healthiest for us.

It is not convenient to have cancer. It is not convenient to have an obese or bulimic child. It is not convenient to waste money on pills and potions in an attempt to replace synthetically the natural, life-giving nutrients we have destroyed through exotic preparation.

Thanks to the food industry's seductive arts, our palates have become so jaded that unless we eat organically, we no longer know what real food tastes like. Meanwhile, our fast foods are taking us ever more swiftly toward an earlier grave. As Michael Pollan observes in his book, *In Defense of Food,* "What people don't eat may matter as much as what they do."

Our nutrition wasn't meant to snap, crackle, and pop, and if food has to be irradiated to be fit to eat we shouldn't be eating it. The function of food is not to titillate our taste buds or bloat our bellies, but to nourish each cell of the complex structure that serves as our only vehicle in this lifetime.

That function is now endangered by genetically engineered food, which deforms the very cells the body needs for healthy development. Those who wish to avoid GE food, the long-term safety of which has yet to be proved, cannot do so unless it is labeled as such. By refusing to label it, the FDA insures that if we are harmed by it, we will be unable to prove the cause—or sue Monsanto.

We, the people, have been betrayed by the very agencies that were created to protect us. It is not surprising the FDA protects the chemical companies, when we learn that most of its regulatory employees come from the pharmaceutical industry or join it when they leave government through the revolving door.

In July of 2009, President Obama appointed former Monsanto lobbyist, Michael Taylor, as a senior adviser to the FDA Commissioner on food safety. Taylor is responsible for the rule that allowed the FDA to ignore evidence that genetically engineered foods (including soy), are very different from natural foods and pose specific health risks.

In his important book, *The Rise of Tyranny*, Jonathan Emord observes:

> FDA political appointees manipulate public resources for the aggrandizement and riches of pharmaceutical companies (and ultimately themselves) at the expense of American liberty, property, and life. They have betrayed the public trust and they have violated the constitution they have sworn an oath to uphold. They have erected a tyrannical bureaucratic oligarchy that sacrifices the lives and property of the many to support the riches of the few.

Thanks to this tyrannical bureaucratic oligarchy, I cannot publicly promote the product that is restoring the hair I lost through chemical poisoning. Vested interests prevailed and the company was put out of business. Thus, a boon for the bald that could benefit millions of men and women cannot be marketed or sold commercially in this Land of the Free, but can be freely purchased outside the United States.

As Benjamin Rush warned us:

> To restrict the art of healing to one class of man and deny privileges to others will constitute the Bastille of medical science.

Welcome to the Bastille.

An Associated Press story in July of 2008 revealed that the FDA has been giving its workers more than $8 million in bonuses to keep them from defecting to pharmaceutical and other regulated industries—this, at a time when the agency is being pressed to spend more money on checking the safety of our food and drugs.

Representative Bart Stupak, Michigan Democrat and chairman of the oversight and investigations subcommittee of the House Committee on Energy and Commerce, remarked, "Congress puts in extra money for food safety, and what does FDA spend it on? Bonuses."

Rep. Stupak might have been even more incensed had he known of some of the agency's expenditures in the 1980s and '90s. Complaining even then that it was underfunded, the FDA spent *sixty million dollars* of taxpayers' money trying to put a cancer-curing doctor out of business.[37] At the same time, newspaper headlines were warning about contaminated fish being served in restaurants, which the FDA claimed it lacked the resources to inspect.

After the agency lost three litigations against Dr. Stanislav Burzynski of Houston Texas, Dr. Burzynski filed a lawsuit against the FDA in May 2007 and won. Since then, he and the agency have enjoyed a fruitful and cooperative relationship.

In recent FDA-monitored clinical trials, for instance, Burzynski achieved remissions of inoperable brain tumors in 116 patients. In addition, the response of 240 patients has been classified as "stable disease." This means that less than 50% of the tumor size remains, with no sign of progression.[38] Why is such good news ignored by the mainstream media?

One case that I followed involved the parents of a baby girl who was born with a tumor wrapped around her brainstem.[39] Told by their oncologist that the glioma was inoperable and the child would not see her first birthday, the distraught parents asked if he knew of any other option they could try. He replied that he did not.

Turning to the Internet, they discovered Dr. Burzynski and applied to him as a last resort. He told them he had never treated a child that young, so he could make no promises, but

---

[37] See *The Burzynski Breakthrough,* by Thomas D. Elias.
[38] Results supplied by the Burzynski Institute.
[39] Inoperable brainstem tumors carry the worst prognosis in the oncology field, but respond well to treatment with Burzynski's antineoplastons.

the baby was given his antineoplastons and the tumor began to shrink.

The parents' medical insurance, however, did not cover unorthodox treatments. When their funds ran low, they begged the insurance company to help with the payments, as it would have done for surgery, chemotherapy, or a bone marrow transplant, all riskier, more painful, and more costly procedures. Because of the child's improvement, their provider agreed—on condition the parents accepted a gag order. They were not to disclose the insurance company's involvement, nor could they speak publicly of the therapy that was saving their baby's life. The company would not even deal directly with Burzynski (paper trails can be risky), but arranged for payment to be made through the parents.

The child is now a healthy, cancer-free nine-year-old, one of many children with inoperable brain tumors whose lives "Dr. B." has saved. Incidentally, her parents later learned their oncologist knew of Burzynski at the time he denied being aware of another option.

For those of us who owe our lives to unorthodox therapies, mistrust of the FDA goes back to 1985, when, in July of that year, its agents entered Dr. Burzynski's clinic, along with the clinics of other alternative practitioners, and seized eleven of his filing cabinets containing past and current patients' medical records, together with all his insurance and billing files.

If one could count the millions of tax-payers' dollars the FDA spent on such raids in the '80s and '90s, the sum would be staggering. Some of the supplement manufacturers who also were raided could not afford the cost of defending themselves and were put out of business—which, of course, was the point.

That the motive behind these raids was not to protect the public, but to protect the pharmaceutical companies and destroy the competition, is shown in a statement from the FDA's own "Dietary Supplements Task Force Final Report," of May 1992:

... to insure that the existence of dietary supplements on the market does not act as a disincentive for drug development.

Raids on alternative therapies intensified after 1990, when David Kessler became commissioner of the agency. Doctors' offices were invaded by Special Weapons and Tactics (SWAT) teams, who confiscated their equipment and patients' confidential files on the pretext that methods were being used which the FDA had not approved. And why had approval been withheld? Not because a single patient had died or been injured—as have thousands on FDA-approved Vioxx and Avandia—but because the legitimate practice of successful drug-free therapies poses an economic threat to big Pharma.

Jonathan Emord describes in his book how, in the 1990s, Kessler refused to allow a proven claim associating folic acid with a reduction in the risk of neural tube defect births to appear on dietary supplements of the product. By disallowing that claim, Kessler—a non-practicing pediatrician—contributed to an estimated 2,500 preventable births *a year* of children born with spina bifida or anencephaly.

As Emord observes:

Since 1990, (FDA) has continued to favor overwhelmingly the suppression of nutrition science over the disclosure of that science.

Kessler, whose medical career has been as an administrator, resigned from the FDA in 1997, claiming a desire to return to private life. In 2003, he was named dean of the School of Medicine and vice chancellor of medical affairs at the University of California San Francisco. In December 2007, he was dismissed under a cloud by the chancellor. He is now a professor at the university.

Forty-five years ago, the FDA was a very different agency. Its finest hour was in 1960 when Frances Kelsey, a newly appointed FDA physician, blocked approval of the drug, thalidomide—already in widespread use in the rest of the world. Bravely resisting pressure from its manufacturer for a swift approval of the drug in the U.S., she refused, because it was suspected of causing Phocomelia.[40]

Thanks to the courage of one woman, America was spared the deformities with which 10,000 children in forty-six other countries were born. Most of the women who took thalidomide escaped giving birth to deformed babies, but in the game of chemical roulette, the odds against escape are growing shorter.

All chemicals should be judged guilty until they are proved innocent.

The AMA and FDA have long practiced a Vatican-like obstruction of progress on behalf of the giant food and pharmaceutical corporations. The AMA was formed in 1847, three years *after* the formation of the American Institute of Homeopathy, which was then the successful, accepted treatment in this country.

As Richard Walters writes in *Options:*

> A trade union of allopathic doctors, the AMA was organized with the undisguised goal of smashing homeopathy in the United States. According to its charter, one of its goals is 'to eliminate the competition, specifically, homeopathy.'
>
> The AMA labeled homeopathy 'a delusion' and stepped up its witch hunt against homeopaths, who were booted out of state medical associations in what the *New York Times,* on June 7, 1873, called 'unjust, unfair,

---

[40] Phocomelia causes babies to be born with shortened or a complete lack of limbs, often with flipper-like appendages for hands, and sometimes feet. Thalidomide, an inadequately tested and potent teratogen, was sold chiefly to pregnant women in the '50s and '60s to combat morning sickness.

and abusive' expulsions. . . . The pharmaceutical industry fully supported the AMA's campaign to destroy homeopathy, well aware that enormous profits could be made from the manufacture and marketing of proprietary medicines. By 1906, all but one medical journal was subsidized by drug companies' advertising, and the allopathic physician in effect became a conscripted sales representative for the pharmaceutical industry.

The ultimate attack on our health freedom, however, is the *Codex Alimentarius,* dubbed "The Food Code" to conceal its purpose (euphemisms are always employed when there is an attempt to hide the truth). Given a Latin name, so that it would not be understood by the public or attract their interest, the Codex Commission—ninety percent of whose delegates are representatives from the multinational pharmaceutical corporations—has been meeting in semi-secrecy in Europe.

Aware of the growing use of alternative methods and the thriving supplement market, the pharmaceutical industry has been trying for years to appropriate its profits through *Codex.* Created in 1962 as a "trade commission" by the United Nations, it was set to become mandatory on December 31, 2009.

In 1997, the German delegation presented a bill titled "Proposed Draft Guidelines for Dietary Supplements," which ruled that *no* vitamin, mineral, herb, etc., can be sold for preventive or therapeutic use. Additionally, none sold as a food can exceed potency levels set by the commission. These dietary supplement restrictions become binding, eliminating the escape clause within GATT [General Agreement on Tariffs and Trade] that allows a nation to set its own standards.

In Germany and Norway, where *Codex* already applies, zinc tablets rose from $4 per bottle to $52, Echinacea rose from $14 to $153, and all such supplements can now be obtained only by prescription. Even vitamin C has been labeled a "drug," and is allowed only by prescription when containing more than 200 milligrams.

Meanwhile, in April of 2007, in one of its many stealth attempts to outlaw alternative modalities, the FDA tried to reclassify all vitamins, supplements and herbs—even *vegetable juices*—as "drugs," to be regulated by its agency. Why does no word of this or of *Codex* appear in the mainstream media? Because *Codex* is the secret child of the pharmaceutical companies, whose sponsorship controls the media's content.

Contrast the crackdown by *Codex* on harmless supplements with the claim of the chemical apologists that fractional amounts of chemicals in our food do not cause us harm. Yet fractions accumulate, interacting with all the other toxins we are exposed to, and with consequences to health that no one can foresee. Add to these all the pharmaceutical and recreational drugs we consume, and it is clear that a growing number of us are becoming toxic time bombs.

"I cannot believe that God plays dice with the Universe," said Einstein, yet this is precisely what the chemical companies are doing with our health—and doing so with a god-like arrogance. I now believe the miscarriage I suffered in 1963 was caused by the chemicals that were accumulating in my body even then. I am certain they caused my breast cancer ten years later, for there is no known incidence of the disease on either side of my birth parents' families. My birth mother died two months short of her 98th birthday after breaking her hip, while the Huestons were long-lived descendents of Scottish crofters.

In 1997, the FDA changed its rules to allow widespread advertising of prescription drugs directly to consumers. These deceitful television ads, accompanied by a soothing pitch man, show smiling actors dancing or playing with children, presumably after taking the product, while a voice-over races through the dangerous side effects at the end. In 2004, the pharmaceutical industry spent over four billion dollars on TV and radio commercials, print ads, and Web-based promotions. Five hundred million dollars was spent on Vioxx alone—the drug that caused thousands of deaths—and, of course, the public pays for these costly ad campaigns in the grossly inflated prices of prescription drugs.

Demand has been growing for a ban on all direct-to-consumer advertising by pharmaceutical companies. Commercials are about suppressing symptoms, not about curing disease, and a drug that relieves your headache may be hiding the cause, which could be food allergy, chemical poisoning or a brain tumor. Acid indigestion and heartburn are the body's way of warning you to change your diet before you try an antacid. A tooth paste will remove the tobacco stains from your teeth, so at least they'll be white while you're dying of lung cancer.

Spoiled by surfeit and strangers to self-denial, we've become a nation addicted to the quick fix: Got a headache, backache, constipation, indigestion, spotty skin, sexual hang-up, anxiety neurosis, smokers' cough, bad breath? Take this pill for instant soothing relief! The American Way of Health. But is health the result? No matter, it beats dealing with the cause, which could mean having to give up something, such as the fat-laden goodies the next commercial will be urging us to buy.

A recent radio commercial listed the drugs a pharmaceutical company has developed for children with cancer, diabetes, hyperactivity, and other ailments. It concluded with the words, "It's the benefits of pharmaceutical research that sustain the hope of Americans for the best in health care." No mention of the side effects of Ritalin, Paxil, Prozac, Zyprexa and other psychotropic drugs. Why are such toxins approved, while safe and successful nutritional cures are termed "controversial" and their efficacy denied?

Unproven cancer drugs, hailed as merely "hopeful," are given prime time publicity on TV, while drug-free therapies that have been curing cancer for years, if discussed at all, receive a segment on an omnibus program, with the final word given invariably to a white-coated debunker.

Reports of cures that are merely "promising" should be prohibited unless they are accompanied by the following information:

Who paid for the research?

What aspect of the study is being withheld?

What specific proof of its claims can be offered *now*— not in animal studies, but in human beings?

In August of 2007, *JAMA* published a study by the Dana-Farber Cancer Institute, which said that cancer patients who eat a diet of red meat, fatty products, refined grains and desserts—a so-called Western diet—may be increasing their chance of disease relapse and early death. The study's lead author, Jeffrey Meyerhardt, MD, MPH, wrote:

> This is the first large observation study to focus on the role of diet in recurrence of the disease. Our results suggest that people treated for locally advanced colon cancer can actively improve their odds of survival by their dietary choices.

Congratulations, Dr. Meyerhardt! It has taken Dana-Farber only seventy years and millions of dollars to discover what Max Gerson discovered in the 1930s. Perhaps it will take only another fifty years to discover that dietary choices can even cure cancer.

Similar to Gerson's Therapy is the program of Dr. Nicholas J. Gonzales in New York City, which also stresses organic nutrition and coffee enemas. His protocol, too, involves enzymes, diet, and detoxification, but differs from Gerson's in that the treatment is tailored to each patient's metabolic type, with fewer juices, and enzymes delivered primarily in supplement form. Although he specializes in pancreatic cancer, Dr. Gonzales has also had success with environmental illness. He, too, has survived attempts by the medical establishment to discredit him.

The belief that only drugs can cure has become so entrenched in the American psyche that when proof of successful *natural* cures is offered, instead of examining the evidence, its legitimacy is denied. "Spontaneous remission" is the explanation offered by oncologists, who grow vague when asked how many such remissions they have seen in their own practice.

Alternative cures are dismissed as "anecdotal evidence" on the basis that only a double-blind, randomized, placebo-controlled study can be relied upon as proof. If that is so, where is the proof that God exists? Or that falling in love is not a self-induced, psychosomatic delusion? (which it may well be). What is the account of Jesus's birth, ministry and resurrection, if not anecdotal? The gospels were written years after his death, and we know how unreliable are witness accounts even an hour after the event.

"Anecdotal evidence," wrote Simon Hoggart, "is the 'experts' sneery way of describing what the rest of us see with our own eyes."

One so-called expert is the radio doctor (formerly an ophthalmologist), who attributes alternative cures to the placebo effect—despite the fact that babies and animals, who are immune to autosuggestion, respond to homeopathic treatment.

Dismissing the evidence for Gulf War Syndrome, chemical sensitivity, silicone breast implant rejection, and the success of unorthodox therapies in general, this non-practicing doctor joined the attack on Dr. Burzynski in the 1990s, parroting the FDA's discredited charges without bothering to check the facts, which he could easily have done with a telephone call to the Burzynski clinic. Of course, by denigrating alternative treatments he keeps his sponsors happy, his listeners in the dark, and his multimillion-dollar lifestyle assured.

A cartoon some years ago showed two doctors walking along the corridor, one saying to the other, *"I have no objection to alternative medicine so long as traditional medical fees are scrupulously maintained."*

Any change of direction will be fought by the doctors and pharmaceutical companies, whose financial control of research into diseases such as cancer gives them monopolistic power. We can sympathize with the doctors, for they have lucrative careers to protect and an expensive education to defend. To admit that some of what they learned in medical school may be out of date—or even wrong—requires a degree of humility not always compatible with their training.

At a Duke University conference on integrative medicine, held in North Carolina in 1999, the editor of the *New England Journal of Medicine,* Marcia Angel, referring to alternative practitioners, stated, "They have an easy time of it, because they're dealing with the worried well."

Actually, no, madam; they're dealing with the abandoned desperate. Millions of people in the U.S. are living in appalling pain, yet in all but thirteen states the law forbids access to the medical marijuana that could relieve their suffering. Some are so desperate they want to die, but the law denies them the right even to this release.

The Death with Dignity Act is about medical care, not drug trafficking, and should not be regulated by the federal government, which forbids cruel and inhuman punishment for the criminal, but condemns the innocent victim of terminal illness to years of unbearable suffering. There is no sanctity of life for those who exist in great pain, if their condition is incurable and they want to put a swift and humane end to their torment. It is beyond sadism to tell someone with motor neuron disease, for example, that the slow shutting down of every bodily function must be endured until, after years of agony, he or she will slowly choke to death.

The British physician, Lord Horder, referring to the Hippocratic Oath, said that while he accepted the fact the physician's duty was to preserve life, it was not his duty to prolong the agony of dying.

Suicide is not a cry for help; it is a cry for release when all hope of help is gone.

Of a recent right-to-die case brought before the U.S. Supreme Court by the State of Oregon, President Bush declared, "Hastening a person's death with drugs is assisted suicide." Quite so. And hastening a person's *unwanted* death with dangerous drugs is legalized murder. Physician-assisted suicide is the compassionate right of a free individual. Denying that right is an act of moral sadism.

We have strayed so far from the ideals that inspired the founders of this country, that when those towering geniuses look down on us now, they must be weeping on Mount Olympus. We are governed by fools, ruled by corporations, lied to by the left as well as the right, and hoodwinked by hypocrisy at every turn. Once the proud Land of the Free and Home of the Brave, America has become the Land of the PAC[41] and Home of the Moral Coward.

Still, it may not be too late if men and women of whatever political hue will heed the oft-misquoted words attributed to the great Irish statesman, Edmund Burke:

> All that is necessary for the forces of evil to win the world is that *enough* good men do nothing.

---

[41] Political action committee.

EPILOGUE

When the Challenger spaceship exploded over the Atlantic Ocean on January 8, 1986, I joined the universal mourning for its gallant crew. Death seems more tragic when those who perish are young and die while embarked on a perilous mission.

Yet, as I watched the shuttle arc crazily into the ocean—its fuel exploding in plumes of smoke against the sky—I found myself grieving as much for the sea and for the future of our planet. The astronauts could have chosen not to risk their lives in a hazardous journey. The creatures of the sea had no such option—nor have those who will eat the fish we are poisoning by our heedless disregard for the earth's fragile ecosystem.

It is a sad truth that no fish is now wholly free of pollution—not even wild salmon, the abundance of which in the market belies its vanishing numbers in the streams. We are committing global suicide on a scale unimagined by Rachel Carson, when she wrote in her seminal book, *The Sea Around Us*:

> It is a curious situation that the sea, from which life first arose, should now be threatened by the activities of one form of that life. But the sea, though changed in a sinister way, will continue to exist; the threat is rather to life itself.

And to aquatic life in particular, as seen in the dying coral reefs, the beached whales and the dolphins flinging themselves onto the shore in the same "mysterious" manner. Having poisoned the habitat of these endearing creatures, we are now destroying their navigating systems with low frequency active sonar testing (LFAS), which pierces their organs and scatters the delicate sensing mechanism on which whales and dolphins rely.

It has been found that when land animals survive with small levels of pesticides in their bodies, they give birth to their young with concentrations strong enough to kill them. Are we running the same risk with our offspring—passing on to them the irreversible breakdown of cell and marrow that we, as adult mammals, have been able thus far to withstand? Children born with strong immune systems may escape for a time, but as toxins proliferate and our food and water become ever more contaminated, the next generation may not be so fortunate.

How many cancers do we need? How many shattered immune systems can we afford before the lethal nature of these poisons is acknowledged and their rampant use curtailed? The evidence is all around us—in the dying fish, the deformed frogs, the disappearing butterflies and bees, and the trees whose branches are denuded by acid rain.

The most urgent question facing us today is not global warming or whether the starving poor of the world can be fed, but whether man's folly will destroy the earth through environmental rapacity, fanatic religious terrorism, or both.

In 1854, Chief Seattle, head of the Suquamish tribe, foreseeing the danger that loomed ahead, observed in his historic speech:

> Where is the thicket? Gone.
> Where is the eagle? Gone.
> The end of living
> And the beginning of survival.

WORKS CONSULTED

Bellini, James. 1989. *High-Tech Holocaust*. David and Charles.

Bishop, Beata. 1996. *A Time to Heal.* 3rd ed. London: First Stone, Penguin Arkana. Available from the Gerson Institute, 1572 Second Ave., San Diego, CA 92101.

Campbell, Joseph. 1976. *The Masks of God,* New York: Penguin Books.

Carson, Rachel. *The Sea Around Us.* Copyright © 1950 by Rachel L. Carson. Reprinted by permission of Frances Collin, Trustee.

Carson, Rachel. *Silent Spring.* Houghton Mifflin. Copyright © 1962 by Rachel L. Carson. Reprinted by permission of Frances Collin, Trustee.

Castaneda, Carlos. 1969. *The Teachings of Don Juan.* Berkeley and Los Angeles: University of California Press.

Cerminara, Gina. 1988. *Many Mansions.* New York: Signet, division of Penguin Group.

Christian Science. 1875. *Science and Health, with Key to the Scriptures.* Boston: Trustees under the Will of Mary Baker G. Eddy.

Cleave, Surgeon-Captain T.L. 1975. *The Saccharine Disease.* Keats Publishing Co. New Canaan, Connecticut.

Coye, Molly. MD, MPH. Spring 1985. "What physicians don't know about occupational exposure to pesticides." *NCAP News.*

Davison, Jaquie. 1977. *Cancer Winner.* Pierce City, MO: Pacific Press.

Davis, Devra. 2007. *The Secret History of the War on Cancer.* New York: Basic Books.

Davis, Lee N. 1984. *The Corporate Alchemists.* Middlesex, Great Britain: Maurice Temple Smith Ltd.

Douglass, William Campbell. August 1997. *Second Opinion.* Atlanta: Second Opinion Publishing, Inc.

Elias, Thomas D. 1997. *The Burzynski Breakthrough.* Los Angeles: General Publishing Group.

Eliot, George. 1874. *Middlemarch,* 2E OWC, edited by David. Carroll (2008), extract of 41 words. By permission of Oxford University Press, 2008.

Emord, Jonathan W. 2008. *The Rise of Tyranny.* Washington, D.C. Sentinel Press.

Erlichman, James. 1986. *Gluttons for Punishment.* England. Peters, Fraser and Dunlop Ltd.

Food and Drug Administration. May 1992*, "FDA vs. The People of the United States, Five years of assault on 'self care.'"*: The Jonathan Wright Legal Defense Fund. Tacoma, Washington.

Gerson, Max. 1958. *A Cancer Therapy: Results of Fifty Cases.* 1st ed. Del Mar, CA: Totality Books.

Hamilton, Edith. 1964. *The Greek Way.* W.W. Norton

Harburg, E.Y. 1965. Poem *"Diagnoses," Rhymes for the Irreverent.* Published by Glocca Morra Music, Administered by Next Decade Entertainment, Inc. All Rights Reserved. Used by Permission. Harburg Foundation.

Hoggart, Simon. October 1991. *The London Observer.*

Journal of the American Medical Association *(JAMA).* Nov. 16, 1946. Volume 132, number 11.

JAMA. 1949. Volume 139, number 2, pp. 93-96.

Korzybski, Alfred. 1933. *Science and Sanity.* Germany: Institute of General Semantics.

LeShan, Lawrence. 1984. *You can Fight for your Life.* M. Evans & Co, Inc., New York.

Mendelsohn, Robert S. MD. 1993. *Immunizations: The terrible Risks Your Children Face That Your Doctor Won't Reveal.* Atlanta: Second Opinion Publishing.

Miller, Neil Z. 1995. *Immunization Theory vs. Reality: Expose on Vaccinations.* Santa Fe: New Atlantean Press.

Piccardi, Giorgio, 1962, *The Chemical Basis of Medical Climatology.* Springfield, Il: Charles C. Thomas, Publisher, Ltd.

Pollan, Michael, 2008. *In Defense of Food.* New York: The Penguin Press.

Randolph, Theron G. Randolph, MD. 1980. *Allergies, Your Hidden Enemy.* New York: Lippincott and Crowell.

Rinkell, Herbert, 1951. *Food Allergy,* University of Michigan: CC Thomas.

Roa Bastos, Augusto, 1986. *I, The Supreme.* English translation. New York: Alfred A. Knopf.

Schlosser, Eric, 2001. *Fast Food Nation: The Dark Side of the all-American Meal.* New York. Houghton Mifflin Company.

Smith, Meg. 1992. "The Burzynski Controversy in the United States and in Canada: a comparative case study in the sociology of alternative medicine." *Canadian Journal of Sociology.* Volume 17, number 2, p. 133.

St. Exupery, Antoine de. 1992. *Wind, Sand and Stars (Terre des Hommes).* Orlando: Harcourt Brace & Co.

Toynbee, Philip. 1988. *End of a Journey.* London: Bloomsbury Publishing Ltd.

Tributsch, Helmut. 1984. *When the Snakes Awake.* Cambridge: MIT Press.

Walters, Richard. 1993. *Options*. Honesdale, PA: Paragon Press.

Watson, Lyall. 1989. *Neophilia.* London: Hodder and Stoughton Ltd. Reproduced by permission of Pollinger Limited and the Estate of Lyall Watson

Watson, Lyall. 1973. *Supernature.* London: Hodder and Stoughton Ltd. Reproduced by permission of Pollinger Limited and the Estate of Lyall Watson.

White, E.B. 1954. *The Points of my Compass.* & 1976, *Letters of E.B. White.* New York, Harper Colophon Books.

White, E.B. 1976, *Essays of E.B. White.* New York, Harper Collins Books.

Wickes, Frances. 1976. *The Inner World of Choice.* Upper Saddle River, NJ: Prentice-Hall, Inc.

www.silentenemy.net